KU-530-379

Contents

Dedications

To Alex, Alice and Fern

Permissions

PasTest would like to thank the following for allowing material to be used in this book:

New England Journal of Medicine
British Medical Journal
British Journal of General Practice
Elsevier Science (The Lancet)

Practice Papers for the MRCGP Written Exam

Dr Rob Daniels MA MRCGP
General Practitioner
Townsend House Medical Centre
Seaton
Devon

Dr Grant Neumegen MBChB MRCGP
General Practitioner (Non-Principal)
Exeter Primary Care Trust
Devon

Dr Joanna Neumegen BM BS BMedSci MRCGP
General Practitioner (Retainer)
St Thomas Medical Group
Cowick Street
Exeter
Devon

Dr Peter Acheson MBChB MRCGP DRCOG
General Practitioner
Claremont Medical Centre
Exmouth Health Centre
Claremont Grove
Exmouth

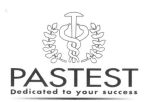

PASTEST
Dedicated to your success

© 2002 PasTest Ltd
Egerton Court
Parkgate Estate
Knutsford
Cheshire WA16 8DX

Telephone: 01565 752000

First edition 2002
Reprinted 2003

ISBN: 1 901198 16 2

A catalogue record for this book is available from the British Library.

The information contained within this book was obtained by the authors from reliable sources. However, while every effort has been made to ensure its accuracy, no responsibility for loss, damage or injury occasioned to any person acting or refraining from action as a result of information contained herein can be accepted by the publisher or the authors.

PasTest Revision Books and Intensive Courses
PasTest has been established in the field of postgraduate medical education since 1972, providing revision books and intensive study courses for doctors preparing for their professional examinations. Books and courses are available for the following specialties:

MRCGP, MRCP Part 1 and Part 2, MRCPCH Part 1 and Part 2, MRCOG, DRCOG, MRCS, MRCPsych, DCH, FRCA and PLAB.

For further details contact:

PasTest Ltd, Freepost, Knutsford, Cheshire, WA16 7BR
Tel: 01565 752000   Fax: 01565 650264
Email: enquiries@pastest.co.uk
Web site: www.pastest.co.uk

Typeset by Vision Typesetting, Manchester
Printed and bound by Bell & Bain Ltd.

Part 1:
Preparation

Introduction

When we decided to write this book we had two goals in mind: firstly, to try to put together a book of practice exam papers, and secondly to attempt to make it useful as a revision aid. After studying for the exam we felt that none of the books available at that time represented the full scope of the exam, and we all found one of the most stressful aspects was trying to get through all the questions in the time allowed. We felt that a book of questions as close to the exam format as possible would allow candidates to practise against the clock and get an idea of how they will cope.

None of the authors are in any way connected with setting the MRCGP exam. We developed these questions by considering everyday problems we have encountered in general practice and creating questions in the MRCGP style from these situations. The hot topics were prompted by our general reading. Our objective was not to give you an insider's view on what will be in the next exam paper, but to show you the type of questions that might be asked and how to approach answering them in a simple format.

As you look through our questions and answers you will notice that there are simple themes which recur in many questions. There is no secret about passing this exam, all you need to do is have a simple framework around which to build your answers. We hope that by looking through our suggestions you will acquire this skill and soon be able to apply it to almost any question you are confronted with.

When you look at our answers, you will probably think that it would be physically impossible for anyone to write that much in 10–20 minutes. That is probably true, but in developing our answers we have tried to expand the points as comprehensively as possible giving enough detail to clearly illustrate the concepts. We hope that this approach will provide a topic revision aid as well as an answer format – the key really is to look at the headings used for each question and use them as a rough template for developing your own answer plans.

Our answers are not perfect, and we are sure you will be able to think of points we have missed. Everyone has their own slant they like to put on an answer, and with practice you will soon develop your own style.

The hot topics questions are derived from current issues we consider to be important and may appear in future papers. There are always more references to find, and you will undoubtedly find those we have missed. The reference lists are for information only. You will not be expected to know page numbers – the publication and year will suffice.

Finally, don't get too worked up over the exam. It is probably the fairest exam you will take in your medical career and if we can manage to get merits in the written paper, so can you. Just stay calm, think things through and you'll find you can tackle any topic thrown at you.

Approach to Hot Topics

The thought of tackling the hot topic section of the exam can be extremely daunting, with a seemingly bottomless pit of areas to cover – try not to panic. You are not expected to have an in-depth knowledge of minute detail, more an appreciation of important current areas affecting everyday general practice.

What is a hot topic? This is difficult to answer but pointers can be gleaned by flicking through the BMJ and BJGP and being aware of topical issues arising from your day-to-day general practice. There frequently seems to be a question based on a recent BJGP editorial, and keeping up to date with topics covered in the 'GP newspapers' can highlight areas to cover. Remember the Paper 1 questions are set months in advance, so don't just consider those topics that are 'hot' close to the exam. Other sources of information include the internet: there are a few good sites, but beware of out of date content.

Of course an easier way to decide what is 'hot' is to buy a book on the subject, e.g. the Pastest Hot Topics book. Many of the exam preparation courses include a session on hot topics, although these can be quite expensive.

If you really enjoy studying hot topics, try summarizing each key paper into one paragraph. Studying for this section in groups rather than individually can lighten the load and provide moral support. Chatting about topics is often a better aid to memory than reading, and knowledge can be pooled.

When approaching revision for these questions, don't try and memorise too many details. The journal and year are more than sufficient. It is much more important to know the crux of the paper's findings rather than the exact reference. An answer plan is not necessary for these questions, but some sort of structure will appeal to the examiners and help you to process your thoughts. Don't be frightened to write down unreferenced points if you can't recall the source; you may still gain points and it isn't negatively marked.

Critical Reading

The best way to prepare for these questions is to practice in small groups. If you are attending a VTS try staying behind for an hour afterwards in the few weeks coming up to the exam. Each week look at a key paper from the hot topics and criticize it as a group. *How to read a paper* by Trish Greenhalgh (BMJ Books, 2000) is probably the best guide to the subject area. Try and come up with a short checklist of points to consider and use this as a reference when analysing a paper.

Don't be fooled into thinking a paper is perfect just because it is in a peer reviewed journal. With a little practice, you'll soon spot the errors.

Answer Plans

The key to passing this paper is not knowing everything about general practice, but rather being able to structure an answer plan thinking broadly of areas to cover. This is much more useful than trying to fathom the examiners' construct. When faced with a question about which you know nothing, don't panic. Write down a list of headings and then go through them systematically with explanatory notes. Once you have done a few you will have the bare bones of a decent answer written down and you are nearly there.

e.g. Mr Smith has come for the results of his blood tests showing he has onchocerciasis. What issues does this raise?

Starting with simple headings you might get:

Consultation Issues

Issues for Mr Smith
Issues for his family
Issues for the doctor
Issues for the practice
Issues for secondary care

Once you have this list, you can start to add to it, e.g.

Consultation Issues

- Explore his ideas, concerns and expectations.
- Be honest about own knowledge and limitations.
- Allow plenty of time for questions.

Issues for Mr Smith

- Effects of treatment – may need time off work, may lose income if no sick pay.
- May want to know more about condition, may search internet and challenge GP with this information.
- May want a second opinion.

And so on. As you can see, quite quickly you can build up a reasonable answer.

Over time, you will develop your own generic answer blueprint. Some people write it down on a piece of paper as soon as they go in to the exam and use it to plan every answer. Some things are quite useful to try and put in every question, e.g. Explore the patient's ideas, concerns and expectations; Give advice about support agencies, etc. Others depend on your own personal style. Don't just write these points, though, as the examiners will want to see that you are not just regurgitating headings but that you can put them into the context of the question you are asked, e.g.

- Explore ideas and concerns – Why has the patient presented to you now? Has he read about this illness in a magazine? Is he worried he will become disabled or lose his job? Does he think he has cancer? Is he considering starting a family and concerned about genetic implications? etc.

Topics to Consider Covering

Here's a general overview of some of the areas to consider covering in a plan – definitely not exhaustive, but hopefully giving some pointers on which you can elaborate.

Approach to Consultation

Rapport, empathy
Ideas, concerns, expectations
Communication skills – cultural/religious consideration
Hidden agendas, assess health belief model
Social/occupational/psychosexual/family context
Ethics: Consent/confidentiality
Autonomy, justice, non-maleficence, beneficience
History
Examination
Investigation: Practice-based/specialist
Management: Check understanding, shared decision making
Safety netting: Follow up, leaflets, good record keeping
Housekeeping: Time management, doctor's feelings/support, e.g. Young Principals group. Educational needs – audit, PLP, mentors

Practice/Wider Issues

Members of primary health care team
Financial/staff implications
Care of colleagues
Professional responsibilities/safety of patients
Local primary care organisation, e.g. PCT
National issues: GP profession – revalidation, morale, recruitment
Government – funding, rationing, service provision

Part 2:
Practice papers

Paper 1

Question 1 See reference material 1.1a, part of a paper entitled 'Meta-analysis of increased dose of inhaled steroid or addition of salmeterol in symptomatic asthma (MIASMA)' (with copyright permission from *British Medical Journal* 320; 1368–1373).

Comment on the outcome measures used

Comment on the methods for identifying suitable studies

Comment on the studies included

Comment on the results shown in Table 5 of reference material 1.1b

Comment on the applicability of these results to clinical practice

Reference material 1.1a

Objective To examine the benefits of adding salmeterol compared with increasing dose of inhaled corticosteroids.
Design Systematic review of randomised, double blind clinical trials. Independent data extraction and validation with summary data from study reports and manuscripts. Fixed and random effects analyses.
Setting EMBASE, Medline, and GlaxoWellcome internal clinical study registers.
Main outcome measures Efficacy and exacerbations.

Methods

Searches

We searched EMBASE, Medline, and GlaxoWellcome databases before the analysis started in January 1998. All publications and abstracts from 1985 onwards in all languages were considered. In a further search in September 1999 we identified no additional studies that fulfilled the search criteria. Study search and selection was conducted by SS.

Selection

Criteria for selection of studies for inclusion in the review were randomised controlled trials; direct comparison between addition of salmeterol to current dose of inhaled steroid and increased (at least doubling) dose of current inhaled steroid for a minimum of 12 weeks; and adults or adolescents (age 12 years or over) with symptomatic asthma on current dose of inhaled steroids.

Quality assessment

All included studies were sponsored by GlaxoWellcome and all met company-wide minimum quality thresholds. All were randomised by using PACT (patient allocation for clinical trials), an in-house, computer based randomisation package validated by the Food and Drug Administration. In all studies, maintenance of the treatment blind was carefully managed with adherence to in-house standard operating procedures. In all studies, treatment packs were supplied numbered in non-identifiable packaging and were dispensed by investigators to the next sequential patient to be randomised in the trial. All studies were conducted according to good clinical practice, and all had received ethical approval. In all studies, appropriate statistical methods were used for summarising and comparing treatments, and methods for handling missing data were preplanned.

Data abstraction

Data abstraction was based on reported summary statistics (means, SD and SE, proportions) for the intention to treat population. Two independent co-workers extracted data from study reports and manuscripts, and their results were compared. Discrepancies were resolved by consensus. Severity of exacerbation was not reported in all studies, and so individual patient datasets were sought and obtained in all but two studies. Severity of exacerbation was assessed independently by two coworkers, without knowledge of treatment allocation or results, who applied the following criteria: severe – requiring oral steroids or admission to hospital; moderate – requiring an increase in inhaled steroid medication; mild – requiring an increase in use of rescue medication.

Quantitative data synthesis

For all measures, treatments were compared each month and for months one to six (when available), with primary interest in the comparisons at three and six months. For peak expiratory flow (recorded by patients twice daily, morning and evening, on diary cards) and forced expiratory volume in one second (FEV1) (recorded at clinic visits) the measure of effect was the difference in means. Previous experience with these measures provided assurance that they have approximately normal distributions. We used reported treatment means or medians for the week or month (as reported) immediately before the next assessment, with previous experience again suggesting approximate normality. For symptoms and use of rescue medication (recorded by the patients on their diary cards) the measure was the difference in the mean percentage of days and nights without symptoms or use of rescue medication. For these measures treatment means were obtained as the mean of the patient means (or medians, as reported), which were calculated over the interval of interest. For exacerbations (recorded in

Reference material 1.1b

Table 5 Numbers (%) of participants with one or more exacerbations of asthma according to severity and difference (95% confidence interval) between treatment with salmeterol and increased dose of inhaled steroid

	Any (mild, moderate, or severe) exacerbation			Moderate or severe exacerbation		
	Salmeterol	Inhaled steroid	Difference	Salmeterol	Inhaled steroid	Difference
Reference						
Greening[2]	78/220 (35)	68/206 (33)	−2.45 (−11.46 to 6.57)	19/220 (9)	18/206 (9)	0.10 (−5.25 to 5.45)
Ind[8]	60/171 (35)	60/165 (36)	1.28 (−8.97 to 11.53)	47/171 (27)	51/165 (31)	3.42 (−6.30 to 13.15)
Woolcock[9]	49/243 (20)	50/251 (20)	−0.24 (−7.31 to 6.82)	40/243 (16)	42/251 (17)	0.27 (−6.29 to 6.84)
Kelsen[10]	37/239 (15)	42/244 (17)	1.73 (−4.86 to 8.33)	18/239 (8)	26/244 (11)	3.12 (−1.99 to 8.24)
Murray[11]	40/260 (15)	44/254 (17)	1.94 (−4.46 to 8.33)	19/260 (11)	31/254 (12)	1.05 (−4.50 to 6.61)
Kalberg[12]	20/246 (8)	32/242 (13)	5.09 (−0.37 to 10.56)	15/246 (6)	27/242 (11)	5.06 (0.09 to 10.03)
Condemi[13]	21/221 (10)	31/216 (14)	4.85 (−1.22 to 10.92)	19/221 (9)	26/216 (12)	3.44 (−2.26 to 9.14)
Van Noord[14]	0/30	2/30 (7)	6.67 (−3.33 to 16.67)	NA	NA	NM
Van Noord[14]	15/109 (14)	13/105 (12)	−1.38 (−10.41 to 7.65)	NA	NA	NM
Vermetten[15]	9/113 (8)	17/120 (14)	6.20 (−1.79 to 14.19)	NA	NA	NM
Pooled results						
Fixed effect			2.73 (0.43 to 5.04)			2.42 (0.24 to 4.60)
Random effects			2.73 (0.43 to 5.04)			2.42 (0.24 to 4.60)
Heterogeneity statistic; df (P value)			5.477; 9 (0.79)			2.687; 6 (0.85)

NA Not applicable: study treatment duration only three months. NM Not measured or available for this study.

case record forms) the measure was the difference in the percentage of participants with one or more exacerbations.

The primary method of combining results was by using a fixed effect model
weighting according to inverse study variance. Random effects estimators were
also calculated to provide an assessment of the degree of heterogeneity.[4] Evidence
for statistical heterogeneity was formally tested and the potential for publication
bias assessed by funnel plot.[7] All analyses were conducted with SAS v6.12.

Your answer . . .

Question 2   An 18-year-old model comes to you complaining of a 3-month history of amenorrhoea.

Outline your management

Question 3   The father of an 8-year-old girl requests that you record and investigate his concerns that his estranged wife may have Munchausen's-by-proxy. What are the implications of this?

Question 4   Mrs Bhatia is having hospital-initiated infertility treatment and attends for a repeat script. You note you wrongly prescribed her clomipramine last time instead of clomiphene. What issues does this raise?

Question 5 **Comment on the following treatments for the menopause, under the headings Factors and Comments and Evidence:**

HRT
SERMs
Phytoestrogens

Your answer . . .

Factors	Comments and Evidence

Factors	Comments and Evidence

Question 6   Your practice is considering setting up a sleep clinic for parents of children with sleep problems. Read reference material 1.2a, an abstract from the paper entitled 'Randomised controlled trial of behavioural infant sleep intervention to improve infant sleep and maternal mood' (with copyright permission from *British Medical Journal* 324; 1062–1065).

Comment on the strengths and weaknesses of the methodology

Comment on the results, shown in reference material 1.2b

Reference material 1.2a

Methods

Participants

This randomised controlled trial was nested within a larger survey. Between May 1998 and April 1999 all mothers attending routine screening sessions for infant hearing at maternal and child health centres in three local government areas in suburban Melbourne, Australia, were invited to complete a survey about their infant's sleep and their own wellbeing (94% response rate). About 80% of children attend these free screening sessions, which are offered to all infants aged 7–9 months.

Survey mothers were eligible for the trial if they reported a problem with their infant's sleep and at least one of the following over the preceding two weeks: waking on more than five nights a week, waking more than three times a night, taking more than 30 minutes to fall asleep, or requiring parental presence to fall asleep. We excluded mothers with insufficient English to complete questionnaires, who were receiving treatment for postnatal depression, or who reported thoughts of self harm and infants with a major medical or developmental problem and those already receiving help for their sleep problem.

Intervention

Mothers in the intervention group attended three private consultations, held fortnightly at their local maternal and child health centre. Sleep management plans were tailored towards individual families. As well as discussing normal sleep cycles, parents were taught that settling after night waking is a learned behaviour that can be modified, infants need to be taught to fall asleep independently, factors reinforcing the sleep problem can be eliminated with appropriate behavioural interventions (see below), an infant's cry may be for more than one reason, and a bedtime routine and consistent daytime naps are desirable.

The main intervention was controlled crying, whereby parents responded to their infant's cry at increasing time intervals, allowing the infant to fall asleep by itself. A few parents chose 'camping out,' whereby they sat with their infant until the infant fell asleep and gradually removed their presence over a period of three weeks. Overnight feeding that contributed to night waking was managed by reducing over seven to 10 days the volume of milk given or time taken to feed. When a dummy was causing problems (needing a parent to find and replace it), parents removed it or attached it to the infant's clothing overnight.

Mothers in the intervention group also received a sleep management plan, information about the development and management of sleep problems, and the same information about normal sleep patterns as the control group. They were asked to maintain daily sleep diaries until the first follow up questionnaire.

Control group

Mothers in the control group were mailed a single sheet describing normal sleep patterns in infants aged 6 to 12 months based on Australian normative data. This sheet did not include advice on how to manage infant sleep problems.

Process

Mothers were randomised to the intervention or control group within two strata ('depressed' and 'not depressed'). Masking occurred at three points (randomisation, data collection, and analysis). Allocation sequences were concealed from researchers and participants until allocation was complete.

We measured outcomes at two months and four months after randomisation by mailed questionnaires. The primary outcomes were maternal report of an infant sleep problem (yes or no) and symptoms of depression measured by the Edinburgh postnatal depression scale with cut off scores of >12 and $\geqslant 10$.

Analysis

We calculated that we would need a sample of 140 women to have an 80% chance of detecting, at a two sided 5% significance level, a three point difference between the two groups in the mean change in the depression score score, with an assumed SD of 4.8 and a loss to follow up of 30%.

We carried out all analyses on an intention to treat basis. Fewer women than anticipated had scores that indicated clinical depression (13 in each group) so we dichotomised depression status at recruitment using community cut off points (depression score <10 and $\geqslant 10$) for analyses.

We used multiple regression models controlling for baseline Edinburgh depression score and allocated group to assess the impact of controlled crying on change in depression scores and factors associated with increased depression scores at two and four months.

Reference material 1.2b

Results

Participant flow and follow up

Of the 738 mothers who completed the survey, 232 were eligible to participate and left contact details and 155 of these agreed to participate.

Sleep

At two months more infant sleep problems had resolved in the intervention group than in the control group (53/76 *v* 36/76, P = 0.005, table 2) and remaining sleep problems were less severe in the intervention group (P = 0.01). In the subgroup of depressed mothers, significantly fewer infants of mothers in the intervention group had a sleep problem at two months (26/33 *v* 13/33, P = 0.001, table 2).

At two months more control mothers than intervention mothers had sought extra help (23/76 (30%) *v* 9/75 (12%), $\chi^2 = 7.54$, P = 0.006) (see also bmj.com). Within the control group more mothers who sought extra help reported that their infant's sleep problem had resolved (13/23 (56%) *v* 23/53 (43(%), $\chi^2 = 1.11$, P = 0.30).

Maternal depression

At two months depression scores fell in both groups, with a slightly greater improvement in the intervention group (table 3). After we controlled for additional professional services, Edinburgh depression score, and allocated group with multiple regression the marginally significant fall in depression scores at two months for the intervention versus control group became significant (point estimate 1.4, 95% confidence interval 0.2 to 2.5, P = 0.02). By four months the greater fall in depression score for intervention mothers was no longer significant, even when we controlled for extra help. For the subgroup of mothers with initial depression scores $\geqslant 10$, scores fell in both groups with a significantly greater improvement in the intervention group at two and four months.

Details of information and strategies that mothers in the intervention group found helpful are given on bmj.com.

Table 2 Number of mothers whose infants' sleep problems had resolved at two and four months for whole sample and subgroups according to mother's Edinburgh depression score

	Resolved at two months			Resolved at four months		
	Intervention	Control	P value*	Intervention	Control	P value*
Whole sample	53/76	36/76	0.005	48/75	39/71	0.26
By Edinburgh score:						
≥10	26/33	13/33	0.001	21/32	14/30	0.13
<10	27/43	22/43	0.34	27/43	25/41	0.86

* χ^2 test.

Table 3 Change in Edinburgh depression scale scores between baseline and two and four months for whole sample and by depression subgroup

	Baseline to two months			Baseline to four months		
	No of women	Change (95% CI)	P* value	No of women	Change (95% CI)	P* value
Whole sample						
Intervention	76	-3.7 (-4.7 to -2.7)	0.06	75	-3.6 (-4.6 to -2.5)	0.45
Control	76	-2.5 (-3.4 to -1.7)		71	-3.0 (-4.0 to -2.1)	
By depression group:						
≥10:						
Intervention	33	-6.0 (-7.5 to -4.0)	0.01	32	-6.5 (-7.9 to -5.1)	0.04
Control	33	-3.7 (-4.9 to -2.6)		30	-4.2 (-5.9 to -2.5)	
<10:						
Intervention	43	-2.0 (-3.1 to -0.8)	0.70	43	-1.4 (-2.6 to -0.2)	0.36
Control	43	-1.6 (-2.7 to -0.5)		41	-2.1 (-3.2 to -1.1)	

* Student's t test.

Question 7 **How could you improve the care of teenagers?**

Question 8   Mr. Green and his wife come to see you for the result of his endoscopy. This showed an inoperable gastric carcinoma. How would you proceed, and what issues would you aim to cover?

Question 9   **Outline your strategies for dealing with difficult patients.**

Question 10 **With regard to end of life decisions, what are the arguments for and against ending life, withdrawing treatment and 'do not resuscitate' orders?**

Question 11 Discuss the evidence regarding the effectiveness of the following interventions in the primary care management of diabetes:

Glitazones
Universal screening
Antihypertensives

Question 12 Read reference material 1.3a, taken from a paper entitled 'A controlled trial of sustained-release bupropion, a nicotine patch, or both for smoking cessation' (*New England Journal of Medicine* 340; 9: 685–692). Copyright © 1999 Massachusetts Medical Society.

Comment on the strengths and weaknesses of the methodology

Comment on the data in Tables 1 and 2 of reference material 1.3b

Reference material 1.3a

Methods

Subjects, screening, and randomization

Subjects were recruited at four study sites by advertisements in the media. The first subject was enrolled in August 1995, and follow-up was completed in March 1997. Of a total of 1182 persons who were screened, 893 met the screening criteria and were enrolled: 218 in Arizona, 227 in California, 220 in Nebraska, and 228 in Wisconsin. The subjects were randomly assigned to one of four treatments with use of an unequal-cell design: 160 subjects were assigned to receive placebo, 244 to receive the nicotine patch, 244 to receive bupropion, and 245 to receive bupropion and the nicotine patch. Randomization was not balanced within sites.

The subjects were screened by means of a telephone interview and a pretreatment session that included a physical examination, electrocardiography, and chest roentgenography. The study protocol was approved by the institutional review board at each site. All participants provided written informed consent.

To be eligible for the study, subjects had to be at least 18 years of age, to smoke at least 15 cigarettes per day, to weigh at least 45.4 kg (100 lb), to be motivated to quit smoking, and to speak English. Only one smoker per household was allowed to enroll in the study. Subjects were excluded for the following reasons: serious or unstable cardiac, renal, hypertensive, pulmonary, endocrine, or neurologic disorders, as assessed by the study-site physician; ulcers; seizure or dermatologic disorders; a current diagnosis of major depressive episode or a history of panic disorder, psychosis, bipolar disorder, or eating disorders; use of a nicotine-replacement therapy within six months before study enrollment; pregnancy or lactation; abuse of alcohol or a non–nicotine-containing drug within the preceding year; use of a psychoactive drug within the week before enrollment; use of an investigational drug within the month before enrollment; prior use of bupropion; current use of other smoking-cessation treatments; and regular use of any non-cigarette tobacco product.

Treatment period

The treatment period was nine weeks. Target quitting dates were set for the second week, usually day 8. Participants were assessed weekly and attended a brief (15 minutes or less) individual counseling session for smoking cessation each week. Counseling topics included motivation, identification of smoking triggers, coping responses, weight management, and use of the medications. The counselors used a standardized treatment developed by Hurt and colleagues. The subjects also received a supportive telephone call from a counselor approximately three days after the target quitting date.

Follow-up period

Follow-up assessments and relapse-prevention counseling occurred during clinic visits 10, 12, 26, and 52 weeks after the start of the study. In addition to clinic visits, subjects received eight telephone calls from a counselor during this period, one per month in months 3, 4, and 5 and 7 to 11. All follow-up counseling was less than 10 minutes in duration per call.

Medications

Subjects in the two bupropion groups received 150-mg tablets of sustained-release bupropion (Zyban, Glaxo Wellcome), and all other subjects received identical-appearing tablets. In the bupropion groups, subjects received 150 mg of bupropion in the morning and a placebo tablet in the evening on days 1, 2, and 3 of treatment; and one bupropion tablet in the morning and one in the evening on days 4 to 63. All other subjects took placebo tablets twice daily from days 1 to 63. Subjects in the nicotine-patch groups used one patch (Habitrol, Novartis Consumer Health) per day for eight weeks beginning on the quitting day (day 8). All other subjects applied a placebo patch each day for eight weeks. The patches used from weeks 2 to 7 each contained 21 mg of nicotine; those used during week 8 each contained 14 mg, and those used during week 9 each contained 7 mg.

Assessments

At base line, serum cotinine, vital signs, and exhaled carbon monoxide were determined; data on smoking history were obtained; and three questionnaires were administered. The portion of the Structured Clinical Interview for the *Diagnostic and Statistical Manual of Mental Disorders,* fourth edition (DSM-IV), concerning mood disorders was used to assess whether subjects had mood disorders. The Beck Depression Inventory assesses the severity of depression. Scores of 0 to 9 are considered to be normal, scores of 10 to 18 indicate mild-to-moderate depression, scores of 19 to 29 indicate moderate-to-severe depression, and scores of 30 to 63 indicate severe depression. The Fagerström Tolerance Questionnaire measures nicotine dependence. Scores can range from 0 to 11, with higher scores indicating more severe dependence.

During the treatment period, vital signs were assessed and the carbon monoxide content of expired air was measured. All subjects were asked to keep a daily diary for the first 12 weeks of the study that included information on smoking status, craving, and withdrawal symptoms. During the follow-up period, the Beck Depression Inventory was given, vital signs and the carbon monoxide content of expired air were measured, and self-reported smoking status was assessed.

Measures of outcome

All 893 subjects were included in analyses of the primary outcome. The primary outcome variable was the point-prevalence rate of abstinence at 6 and 12 months of follow-up. Subjects were considered to be abstinent if they reported not smoking since the preceding clinic visit and had an expired carbon monoxide concentration of 10 ppm or less. Subjects were considered to be continuously abstinent if they had not smoked after the quitting day, as confirmed by a carbon monoxide concentration of 10 ppm or less at all clinic visits during the 12-month study. Secondary outcome measures included withdrawal symptoms, body weight, and Beck Depression Inventory scores.

Statistical analysis

Chi-square and analysis of variance were used to test for base-line differences in demographic and smoking-history variables. All statistical tests were two-sided and had an alpha level of 0.05. Sample sizes were based on the results of a previous study of bupropion in which the abstinence rates at four weeks were 40 percent in the bupropion group and 24 percent in the placebo group. We estimated that 130 subjects were needed in the placebo group and 230 subjects were needed in the treatment groups for the study to have a power of 0.80 to detect such a difference at an alpha level of 0.05. All subjects who discontinued treatment early or who were lost to follow-up were classified as smokers.

Logistic-regression analysis was used to determine pairwise differences among groups in the abstinence rates. The Kaplan–Meier method was used to analyze differences in rates of continuous abstinence; homogeneity among treatments and pairwise differences were tested with the log-rank test.

Withdrawal symptoms were assessed daily with a composite score calculated as the mean of eight items in the daily diary: craving for cigarettes; restlessness; increased appetite; depressed mood; anxiety; difficulty concentrating; irritability, frustration, or anger; and difficulty sleeping (DSM-IV symptoms plus craving). The severity of each symptom was rated on a five-point scale, as absent (0), slight (1), mild (2), moderate (3), or severe (4). Repeated-measures analysis of variance was used to analyze the change in scores from base line (before smoking cessation) to after smoking cessation. Group coding was used that permitted tests of the independent and interactive effects of the two pharmacotherapies. In one analysis, the changes in scores during the first six days after the quitting date were analyzed; in a second analysis, the changes in scores during each week of the eight-week period after the quitting date were analyzed. To control experiment-wise error, Tukey's studentized range test was used for pairwise group comparisons of changes in scores that were found to be significantly different; this same strategy was used to analyze body weight and Beck Depression Inventory scores. Adverse events that began or increased during the treatment phase were coded with COSTART (Coding Symbols for Thesaurus of Adverse Reaction Terms), and differences between groups were tested by Fisher's exact test.

Reference material 1.3b

Table 1 Base-line characteristics of the subjects*

Characteristic	Placebo (N = 160)	Nicotene patch (N = 244)	Bupropion (N = 244)	Nicotine patch and bupropion (N = 245)
Age (yr)	42.7 ± 10.2	44.0 ± 10.9	42.3 ± 10.2	43.9 ± 11.6
Female sex (%)	58.8	51.6	51.6	49.4
White race (%)	93.1	93.0	93.9	92.2
Weight (kg)	74.2 ± 14.6	76.9 ± 17.4	76.5 ± 16.2	76.1 ± 16.1
Education (%)				
High-school graduate or less	24.4	21.3	21.3	18.4
Some education after high school	48.1	51.2	46.3	48.6
College graduate or more	27.5	27.5	32.4	33.1
No. of cigarettes smoked daily	28.1 ± 10.6	26.5 ± 9.4	25.5 ± 8.8	26.8 ± 9.4
Years of smoking cigarettes	25.6 ± 9.9	26.8 ± 11.1	24.6 ± 10.5	26.7 ± 11.6
No. of previous attempts to quit	2.8 ± 3.0	2.7 ± 2.4	3.1 ± 4.7	2.5 ± 2.4
Expired carbon monoxide (ppm)	30.2 ± 12.2	28.3 ± 9.9	28.4 ± 11.1	28.7 ± 11.1
Serum cotinine (ng/ml)	358 ± 157	373 ± 204	357 ± 170	362 ± 165
Fagerström score†	7.5 ± 1.8	7.4 ± 1.7	7.4 ± 1.6	7.3 ± 1.8
Other smokers in household (%)	37.1	28.3	28.7	24.5
Previous use of nicotine patch (%)	36.5	38.1	36.9	34.7
Previous use of nicotine gum (%)	34.0	23.4	28.3	28.2
History of major depression (%)‡	15.6	18.0	20.9	17.6
Beck Depression Inventory score§	4.0 ± 4.4	3.9 ± 4.5	4.4 ± 5.1	3.5 ± 4.7

*Plus–minus values are means ± SD. Percentages do not all sum to 100, because of rounding.
†The range for the Fagerström Tolerance Questionnaire score is 0 to 11, with scores of 6 or greater indicating higher levels of nicotine dependence.
‡History of major depression was assessed by the Structured Clinical Interview, for the DSM-IV. Persons meeting criteria for a current diagnosis of major depression were excluded from the study.
§The scores on the Beck Depression Inventory can range from 0 to 63, with scores of 0 to 9 considered to be within the normal range. Scores of 10 to 18 indicate mild-to-moderate depression, scores of 19 to 29 moderate-to-severe depression, and scores of 30 or higher severe depression.

Your answer . . .

Table 2 Primary efficacy outcomes*

Outcome	Placebo (N = 160)	Nicotine patch (N = 244)	Bupropion (N = 244)	Bupropion and nicotine patch (N = 245)
No. evaluated at 6 mo	86	159	178	195
Abstinence at 6 mo – % (no.)	18.8 (30)	21.3 (52)	34.8 (85)	38.8 (95)
Odds ratio (95% CI)	–	1.2 (0.7–1.9)	2.3 (1.4–3.7)	2.7 (1.7–4.4)
P value				
For the comparison with placebo	–	0.53	<0.001	<0.001
For the comparison with patch	–	–	0.001	<0.001
For the comparison with bupropion alone	–	–	–	0.37
No. evaluated at 12 mo	82	152	169	181
Abstinence at 12 mo – % (no.)	15.6 (25)	16.4 (40)	30.3 (74)	35.5 (87)
Odds ratio (95% CI)	–	1.1 (0.6–1.8)	2.3 (1.4–3.9)	3.0 (1.8–4.9)
P value				
For the comparison with placebo	–	0.84	<0.001	<0.001
For the comparison with patch	–	–	<0.001	<0.001
For the comparison with bupropion alone	–	–	–	0.22

* Point-prevalence rates of abstinence based on biochemically confirmed (by an expired carbon monoxide concentration of $\leqslant 10$ ppm) self-report of abstinence during the seven days preceding assessment of smoking status at a given time. The treatment period was nine weeks. Odds ratios were computed by logistic-regression analysis, which was used to determine pairwise differences in abstinence rates. Subjects who discontinued treatment or were lost to follow-up before a visit were classified as smokers for that visit. CI denotes confidence interval.

Paper 2

Question 1 A 45-year-old businessman consults you because he has problems getting an erection. Discuss your management.

Question 2   'You can't teach an old dog new tricks.' How can GPs stay up-to-date, and what are the risks and benefits of this?

Question 3   A 45-year-old secretary complains of intermittent loss of sensation in her left hand. You know her father has multiple sclerosis. How would you proceed?

Question 4   **Discuss the use of referral rates in general practice with reference to the literature.**

Question 5   The senior partner in your practice has the largest prescribing bill in the health authority. What are the implications of this and how would you approach the situation?

Question 6   A 41-year-old ex-serviceman asks for help. He complains of
palpitations, nightmares and work difficulties. He smells of alcohol.
His wife has seen you about relationship difficulties. Outline your
approach to this problem.

Question 7   Your practice is considering providing a complementary medicine service to your patients. You wish to make the decision evidence-based. What are the difficulties in researching complementary therapies such as acupuncture? Comment under the headings below:

Study design
Bias and confounding
Results

Question 8   See reference material 2.1a, taken from the paper 'A single blind trial of reflexology for irritable bowel syndrome' (with copyright permission from *British Journal of General Practice* 2002; 52: 19–23).

Comment on the strengths and weaknesses of the methodology

Comment on the results shown in reference material 2.1b

Reference material 2.1a

Method

The research was conducted in a single geographical area of a city in the north of England during 1999. After full consideration of methodological debates surrounding CAM research, it was designed as a single-blind trial. Four general practices were used; all served predominantly white patients.

Tight inclusion criteria were employed. These were:
Patients currently under the care of a primary care physician following referral to a gastroenterologist;
Diagnosis of IBS in line with the Rome Criteria; and, therefore, the exclusion of other causes of symptoms.

One exclusion criterion previous use of reflexology,was used. The purpose of this approach was threefold. First, to ensure that the IBS classification was as standard as possible from patient to patient and that symptoms were not caused by other conditions. Secondly, to ensure that participants were chronic sufferers, thereby minimising the potential for spontaneous symptom remission or for symptom reduction owing to increased attention alone. Thirdly, the exclusion criterion was employed to ensure that patients would be unable to distinguish between treatment and control groups. Written consent from participants, and ethical approval from a Local Ethics Committee, were sought and received.

Participants, identified via a notes search, were initially contacted by their GP and then by the researcher. Ninety per cent of those sent full details agreed to participate. All were currently under the care of their GP following secondary care referral.

Patients were randomised to one of two groups;

Reflexology group. Treatment consisted of six (four weekly and two fortnightly) 30-minute sessions conducted as close as possible to 'normal' practice.

Indistinguishable control group. As benefits of CAM are frequently dismissed as the result of increased contact alone, the main aim was to control for that contact. This group were exposed to exactly the same number of contact sessions as the experimental group. Sessions were carried out in exactly the same way, following the same procedures, with the single exception of a

nonreflexology foot massage was given (a massage that did not include the application of pressure on key points of the feet that is characteristic of reflexology). According to reflexology theory this should have no curative effect as no stimulation of healing has occurred.

All sessions were conducted in the participants' surgery. 'Holistic' features of a standard consultation, such as lifestyle advice, were excluded from the procedure. This was because it can be argued that the fundamental validity of reflexology rests on the extent to which its specific form of foot massage produces an impact a discernible change unrelated either to the process of consulting or to behavioural change. The study's lead reflexologist was consulted throughout to minimise grounds for the *post hoc* rejection of findings by advocates of reflexology on the basis of the inappropriateness or artificiality of project design. A written code of conduct, refined during pilot work with two people from outside of the trial, was followed to maximise procedural rigour.

Randomisation by alternation was used. Participants were recruited practice by practice since, given the small numbers involved in each practice, full randomisation in these small blocks would have been impractical.

A Health Assessment Sheet, similar to those used successfully in other IBS trials, was used to provide a quick and easy means for participants to record symptom intensity. The defining symptoms of IBS – abdominal pain and constipation/diarrhoea, plus bloatedness/abdominal distention, were assessed daily on a five-point (0 to 4) scale. The forms were completed by all participants for two weeks before the first session (details of sessions below), throughout the intervention, for two weeks after, and again for two weeks at follow-up three months after the final session. Results are based on a comparison of symptoms at baseline: end of Week 2 (prior to the first session), and outcome: Week 10 (after the last session). Follow-up data were based on a comparison of symptom intensity at baseline with symptom intensity three months after the end of the intervention. There was an 80% power (aiming at 18 patients per arm), with 5% significance to detect a difference of 50% of controls and 90% of the experimental group achieving health improvement on the principal outcome measure (abdominal pain). As no published evidence existed in the area, the figures resulted from an assessment of the kind of difference that would be regarded as clinically significant (and from clinical experience might be anticipated), i.e., the kind of difference that might underpin integration into mainstream practice. Data were analysed using a Mann–Whitney U test.

Reference material 2.1b

Results

Thirty-four patients (28 female, six male, mean age = 48, age range = 19 to 72) a number larger than in much of the related work on IBS and CAM[142] – completed the study. Symptom duration ranged from 18 months to 15 years. Baseline depression was negligible (mean = 3.6, Hospital Anxiety and Depression Scale [HAD]), baseline anxiety was higher (mean = 9.6 HAD, (7 to 10 indicates mild anxiety, 11 to 14 indicates moderate anxiety). The intervention was completed by 19 participants in the reflexology group (15 at the three-month follow-up) and 15 in the control group (13 at the three-month follow-up).

There were no significant differences in baseline characteristics between the two groups (abdominal pain: reflexology – median = 1.4, interquartile range (OR) = 0.6 to 21, control – median = 0.7, IQR = 0.5 to 1.3; constipation/diarrhoea: reflexology median = 1.9, (OR = 1.2 to 2.1, control – median = 1.2, IQR = 0.3 to 1.7; bloatedness: reflexology median = 2.5, (OR = 1 .3 to 3.1, control – median = 2.0, (OR = 1.0 to 2.2).

Fifteen participants were approached at varying stages of the trial and asked if they could confidently identify which group they belonged to. None expressed a 'confident' assessment although two offered a 'guess' and both of these guesses were correct. A reasonable degree of confidence that the blind nature of the trial was maintained can therefore be expressed.

Abdominal pain

Abdominal pain is the principal outcome measure and one of the key defining symptoms of IBS laid out in the Rome Criteria. These data show no significant difference between the impact of reflexology and control on this symptom (control – median = −0.40, (OR = −0.90 to 0.00, n = 15; reflexology – median = −0.10, (OR = −0.80 to 0.10, n = 19; U = 114.0, P = 0.32; Figure 2). No change in outcome was recorded at the three-month follow-up (control – median = −0.25, reflexology - median = 0.00).

Constipation/diarrhoea

This is the second variable drawn from the Rome Criteria for IBS. Again, there is no evidence of any difference between the groups (Figure 3), and on this measure very little impact was recorded at alt (control – median = −0.30, IQR = −0.80 to 0.20, n = 15; reflexology median = 0.05, IQR = −0.53 to 0.43, n = 18; U = 115.0, P = 0.47). This was confirmed at follow-up (control median = 0.00; reflexology – median = 0.10).

Bloatedness

The pattern established with the first two symptoms is repeated with bloatedness (Figure 4) (control – median =−0.40, IQR = −1.05 to −0.15, n = 13; reflexology – median =−0.10, IQR = −0.60 to 0.20, n = 17; U = 77.5, P = 0.17.

Again, these results were confirmed at follow-up (control median = −0.42; reflexology median = −0.10).

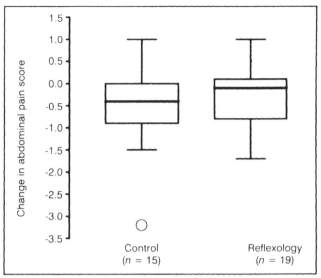

Figure 2. Change in abdominal pain score at end of intervention.
Key: ☐ IQR; ——median; ⊢——⊣ all data excluding outliers; ○ outliers
(> 1.5 x IQR from the edge of the box).

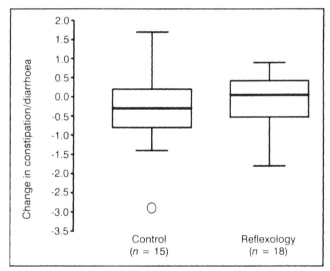

Figure 3. Change in constipation/diarrhoea at end of intervention.
Key: ☐ IQR; ——median; ⊢——⊣ all data excluding outliers; ○ outliers
(> 1.5 x IQR from the edge of the box).

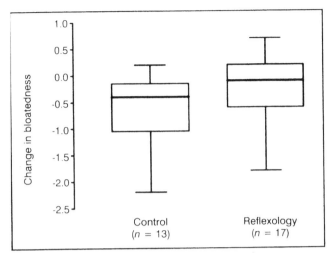

Figure 4. Change in bloatedness at end of intervention.
Key: ☐ IQR; ── median; ⊢──┤ all data excluding outliers; ◯ outliers
(> 1.5 x IQR from the edge of the box).

Question 9   **Your practice is considering becoming paperless. What considerations may surround this decision?**

Question 10 A 38-year-old with knee pain informs you during the consultation that her husband is clinical director of the local hospital. What considerations affect the consultation, and how would you proceed?

Question 11 **What are the challenges in managing dyspepsia? Discuss the evidence under the headings below:**

Investigations
Treatment

Question 12 Personal Medical Services (PMS) or General Medical Services (GMS)? Discuss the pros and cons of the contractual options for general practice.

Paper 3

Question 1 See reference material 3.1a, an extract from 'Survival outcome of care by specialist surgeons in breast cancer: a study of 3786 patients in the west of Scotland' (with copyright permission from *British Medical Journal* 1996; 312: 145–148).

Comment on the design of the study

Comment on the results in table 1 (reference material 3.1b)

Give possible alternative explanations

Reference material 3.1a

Patients and methods

We identified all patients with breast cancer aged under 75 years whose disease was recorded in the west of Scotland cancer registry as histologically verified and who lived in a geographically defined area between 1 January 1980 and 30 June 1988 (when the United Kingdom national breast screening programme began locally).

The study population was defined by identifying the postcode sectors that formed the natural catchment areas for each of 10 hospitals concerned, which remain anonymous for reasons of confidentiality.

This procedure produced a population base of 1.5 million and 3786 histologically verified cases of breast cancer in women. We were unable to find the pathology records for only 2% of cases. Cases which were not histologically verified were excluded from the study. Of patients with breast cancer within the study area, 89% or more were treated at their local hospital. The pathology departments of all hospitals in the study area gave access to their data on tumour size and nodal involvement. Histological grade was available from only two of the 10 hospitals studied and applied to 412 patients from these.

The specialist surgeons were chosen by local perception. Over the time period of the study they each demonstrated the following indicators of specialist interest. These were setting up of a dedicated breast clinic; a defined association with pathologists and oncologists; organising and facilitating clinical trials; and maintaining a separate record of all patients with breast cancer in their care.

They kindly supplied the names of all patients in the care of their teams within the time period 1980 to mid-1988. A total of 918 patients were categorised in this way. The 2868 remaining patients were considered to have received non-specialist care. An independent scrutiny of surgeons' names on the pathology reports confirmed that the names of the patients supplied by the specialists were accurate and complete. We also confirmed that the remaining patients were indeed cared for by those categorised as non-specialists. The names of the non-specialists in the hospitals studied were not abstracted. Survival of all patients up to the end of 1993 was ascertained from death certificates provided by the registrar general (Scotland) to the cancer registration system. Information on socioeconomic status was derived for the postcode sectors included in the study area by using the Carstairs deprivation index.

We carried out an initial analysis of survival outcome with adjustment for prognostic factors – age (entered as a continuous variable), deprivation category (as three separate categories), and tumour size (as three separate categories) but not nodal involvement – using Cox's proportional hazards model. An additional analysis was carried out that included nodal involvement as a prognostic factor with the categories node negative (based on four or more nodes sampled), node negative (based on one to three nodes sampled), and node positive. This took account of concern about the comparability of nodal information for patients cared for by specialists and non-specialists. Tumour size and the state of the nodes were used in preference to conventional staging as they provide a more precise measure of prognosis for an individual patient.

Reference material 3.1b

Table 1 Survival in women with breast cancer according to whether they were treated by surgeon with specialist interest

Detail	Surgeons with specialist interest	Surgeons with no specialist interest	All patients
No of women	918	2868	3786
Percentage (SE) surviving at 5 years	67% (1.6%)	58% (0.9%)	60% (0.8%)
Percentage (SE) surviving at 10 years	49% (1.9%)	41% (1.0%)	43% (0.9%)
Relative hazard ratio (95% confidence interval) adjusted for age, deprivation, and tumour size	0.83 (0.74 to 0.92)	1.0 (baseline)	
Relative hazard ratio (95% confidence interval) adjusted for age, deprivation, tumour size, and nodal involvement	0.84 (0.75 to 0.94)	1.0 (baseline)	

Question 2   **A concerned father brings his 14-year-old son asking you to screen him for drugs. Discuss the issues this raises.**

Question 3   A 33-year-old man asks to be referred for a circumcision, informing you this was suggested after a consultation over the internet for premature ejaculation. Outline your management of this consultation.

Question 4   **A hostel for the homeless is to be opened in your practice area. With reference to the literature, comment on the following areas of care for these patients, under the headings Factors and Comments and Evidence:**

Barriers to care
Medical problems
Provision of care

Your answer . . .

Factors	Comments and Evidence

Factors	Comments and Evidence

Question 5 A 15-year-old girl complains of problems 'down below'. What issues surround this consultation?

Question 6   A 48-year-old woman asks for a repeat thyroxine script, started
recently for weight loss by one of your partners. Her BMI is 26 and
no thyroid blood tests are recorded. How do you manage this
request?

Question 7   **What are the difficulties in dealing with doctors as patients?**

Question 8   You are a member of a working party carrying out a review of
community care of patients with Parkinson's disease. You are keen
to make any decisions evidence-based.

Outline how you would gather your evidence

Details of the methodology of one paper being discussed ('Effects of
community based nurses specializing in Parkinson's disease on
health outcomes and costs: randomized controlled trial', *British
Medical Journal* 324; 1072–1075) are given in reference material
3.2a. With copyright permission from the BMJ.

Comment on the strengths and weaknesses of the study design,
intervention and sampling methods

Reference material 3.2a

Methods

Recruitment

Our sampling frame included all English health authorities coterminous with
local authorities in 1995 that did not already have well developed community
based services of nurse specialists in Parkinson's disease. After random selection,
we recruited nine health authorities (see bmj.com).

We approached all the general practices in the nine areas and asked them to
identify patients with a diagnosis of Parkinson's disease from their doctor or
hospital. Eligible patients were those taking one or more antiparkinsonian drugs.
They were invited to take part by letter from either their doctor or us. We
excluded patients aged 17 years or less or those with severe mental illness or
cognitive impairment sufficient (in the view of their doctor) to preclude valid
informed consent

Statistical power and randomisation

With an expected dropout rate of 15% in each year of the trial, we determined a
total initial sample size of 1600 patients could detect a 10% change in a categorical
outcome having an initial prevalence of 50%, with 80% power at the 5% significance level. Patients were randomised within practice by using block randomisation lists that reflected the randomisation ratio of the health authority area (see
bmj.com).

Nurse intervention

Nine nurses were employed by the university and trained at the Nursing and
Midwifery School, University of Sheffield. They completed a course on meeting
the special needs of people with Parkinson's disease and their carers. In the trial

their clinical position in the community was advisory to the general practitioner rather than clinically autonomous. Each nurse was supplied with a leased car and a mobile phone and assumed areas of responsibility (box) under the guidance of a nurse manager. Their working pattern was characterised by a time use study in which the nurses kept a diary of their daily work over two one week periods. Patients in the control group were not provided with additional services until the end of the two year intervention, when they were offered one assessment from a nurse specialist.

Baseline and follow-up assessments

Trained lay interviewers collected information relevant to health outcome and costs at baseline and at one and two years. Before each interview the patients were sent a questionnaire eliciting information about self perceived health status.

Self-completed questionnaire

The questionnaire included a validated instrument for measuring the functioning and wellbeing of patients with Parkinson's disease, the PDQ-39, and the Euroqol, a health related quality of life measure. The questionnaires at one and two years also included a self perceived global health question asking patients about change in their general health over the preceding 12 months. This question is used by clinicians specialising in Parkinson's disease to gauge patient perception of changes in wellbeing between visits to hospital clinics. The five possible responses to this question were much better (score 0), better (1), same (2), worse (3), and much worse (4). Because the response in the second year depends on the response in the first year, a score was derived representing an individual's change in health over the two year period (see bmj.com). The score ranged from 0 (best) to 8 (worst).

Interviews

Face to face interviews covered three broad groups of questions: assessment of clinical outcome measures, use of health and social services, and personal characteristics. Clinical assessment included questions relating to duration and severity of disease and a test of patients' ability to put dots in a grid of 90 squares within 30 seconds (dot in square test). The Columbian rating scale was used to test patients' ability to rise from a chair with a hard seat to allow 'push off.' Adverse events such as fractures were also recorded.

Costs

Services, aids, and adaptations to the home were valued by using data compiled by the Personal Social Services Research Unit and priced at 1996 Costs; drugs were priced from the *Monthly Index of Medical Specialities* 1996 net ingredient costs. For all these elements average costs were calculated by summing the unit cost per patient, annualising where appropriate, and dividing the total by the number of patients in the study. Costs incurred by carers are not reported here.

The interviews were repeated at one and two years. Follow up of mortality continued for 4 years (to 31 December 1999).

Statistical analysis

We estimated between group differences using ordinal logistic regression for progression on stand-up test, logistic regression for bone fracture, ordinary linear regression for dot in square scores and quality of life measures, and Cox regression for mortality. For each patient we calculated the changes in healthcare cost (excluding costs for carer and social security benefit) over the two years.

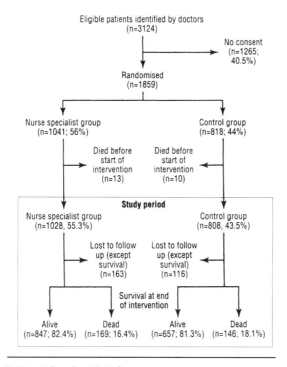

Participant flow through study

Question 9   Extracts from the results of the paper entitled 'Effects of community based nurses specializing in Parkinson's disease on health outcomes and costs: randomized controlled trial' (*British Medical Journal* 2002; 324: 1072–1075) are given in reference material 3.3a. With copyright permission from BMJ.

How do the results support a decision in favour of the intervention?

How do the presented results support a decision against the intervention?

Comment on the analysis of the costs

Are there any other explanations for the lack of effect in the results?

Reference material 3.3a

Results

Participant flow and follow-up

Of the 863 eligible practices, 438 (51 %) agreed to participate and 1859 patients with Parkinson's disease were randomised (figure). No noticeable differences were observed between treatment groups at baseline (table 1).

At the end of the study, patients showed a decline in health status (see bmj.com). The average self perceived health score as assessed by the global health question was 4.89, another indicator of deterioration; unchanged self perceived health over 2 years would score 4 on this question.

Primary outcomes

Objective measures of health

At two years' follow up the severity of Parkinson's disease, the proportion of each group sustaining a fracture, and mortality was not significantly different between the two groups (table 2).

Patient wellbeing

No differences were observed in Euroqol scores or in any dimension of the PDQ-39 at the end of the study (see bmj.com). However, when the patients were asked about change in general health in the global health question, the combined scores from years 1 and 2 differed between groups, with the nurse group doing significantly better than the control group (difference in means −0.23, 95% confidence interval −0.4 to −0.06).

Costs

The mean annual cost among the nurse group increased from £4050 in the year preceding the study to £5860 in the second year of the study and from £3480 to £5630 among the control group, the difference in mean increase between groups not being significant (table 3). The mean costs of different components of health care were also similar in each group during the second year; the provision of nurse specialist care cost £200 per patient per year.

Nurse activity

The time use study showed that the nurse specialists assessed an average of 14 patients per week, 75% at home, 14% at general practices, and 11% in hospital consultant clinics. Patients in the nurse group received on average eight assessments by the nurse per year. In a typical week the nurses made five visits to general practitioners, two to carers, and one to a consultant to discuss patient care. Apart from face to face contact, considerable amounts of nurse time were spent each week on administration, letter writing, telephoning patients (6 hours), and travelling (8.4 hours).

Reference material 3.3a (continued)

Table 1 Characteristics of participants at beginning of study, by treatment group. Values are numbers (percentages) unless stated otherwise

	Nurse group (n=1028)	Control group (n=808)
Sociodemographic characteristics		
Age (years):		
<70	354 (34.4)	256 (31.7)
70–77	359 (34.9)	290 (35.9)
>77	315 (30.6)	262 (32.4)
Male	588 (57.2)	456 (56.4)
Accommodation:		
Free living	916 (89.1)	716 (88.6)
Sheltered	47 (4.6)	41 (5.1)
Institution	65 (6.3)	51 (6.3)
Free living, with main carer	631 (61.4)	489 (60.5)
Manual social class	462 (44.9)	382 (47.3)
Health measures		
Years since diagnosis*:		
0–4	517 (50.3)	400 (49.5)
5–9	211 (20.5)	183 (22.6)
>9	247 (24.0)	187 (23.1)
Stand-up group†:		
1, no problems	453 (46)	344 (42.6)
2, without holding on	187 (18.2)	155 (19.2)
3, unable or had to hold on	353 (34.3)	299 (37.0)
Bone fracture in past 12 months	55 (5.4)	50 (6.2)
Mean (SD) best hand score‡	45.6 (21.7)	45.0 (21.8)
Drugs:		
Levodopa	869 (84.5)	695 (86.0)
Levodopa and anticholinergic	98 (9.5)	62 (7.7)
Levodopa and dopamine agonist	84 (8.2)	45 (5.6)
Levodopa (mg daily), median (quartiles)	300 (150, 550)	300 (150, 500)
Mean (SD) Euroqol score	0.43 (0.35)	0.43 (0.36)
Mean (SD) PDQ-39 summary score	37.9 (21.8)	38.2 (21.8)

* Missing data as some patients unaware of time since diagnosis.
† Missing data as some patients refused test.
‡ Dot in square test.

Table 2 Clinical outcomes at end of study. Values are numbers (percentages) unless stated otherwise

	Nurse group (n=696)	Control group (n=558)	Odds ratio (95% CI) (nurse v control)	P value
Stand-up group*:				
1, no problems	248 (35.6)	221 (39.6)	1.15 (0.93 to 1.42)	0.19
2, without holding on	114 (16.4)	82 (14.7)		
3, unable or had to hold on	329 (47.3)	247 (44.3)		
Bone fracture during study	92 (13.2)	62 (11.1)	1.20 (0.85 to 1.69)	0.31
Mean (SD) best hand score†	45.3 (21.2)	46.0 (21.1)	−0.70 (−3.25 to 1.84)‡	0.59
Mortality:	(n=1016)	(n=803)		
Died by 1 January 1998 (2 years)	169 (16.6)	146 (18.2)	0.91 (0.73 to 1.13)§	0.38
Died by 1 January 2000 (4 years)	353 (34.7)	307 (38.2)	0.89 (0.76 to 1.03)§	0.12

* Missing data as some patients refused test.
† Dot in square test.
‡ Regression coefficient and confidence interval from linear regression model.
§ Hazard ratio.

Table 3 NHS and local authority costs (in £000s), excluding benefits. Values are mean (maximum)

	Nurse group (n=1028)	Control group (n=808)
Year preceding study*	4.05 (55.4)	3.48 (35.0)
Year 2†	5.86 (39.1)	5.63 (33.1)
Individual mean increase†	2.54 (34.6)	2.80 (31.6)‡
Cost components in year 2†		
Nurse specialist	0.20	
Institutional cost	2.86 (20.6)	3.31 (20.6)
Respite care	0.09 (12.8)	0.08 (7.98)
Hospital cost	0.79 (17.9)	0.74 (22.3)
Primary health care	0.15 (6.34)	0.19 (6.34)
Therapy	0.10 (4.33)	0.10 (4.71)
Drugs§	0.70 (25.3)	1.12 (3.74)
Home help	0.34 (2.50)	0.30 (2.50)

* All patients entering study.
† Patients at end of study.
‡ P value 0.47 (difference −0.26, −0.98 to 0.45) (unpaired t test with unequal variances). P value and 95% confidence interval checked with 2000 bootstrapped samples.
§ Excludes apomorphine.

Question 10 You see a 55-year-old woman who works in a pottery with her husband. She tells you she has been seen at the walk-in centre, who told her that she should be referred to the allergy clinic regarding a rash. What issues does this raise, and how would you proceed?

Question 11 **Osteoporosis is a significant problem. For each of the three parts to the question, write your answers in separate columns under the headings Factors and Comments and Evidence:**

Prevention of osteoporosis
Prevention of fracture
Treatment

Your answer . . .

Factors	Comments and Evidence

Factors	Comments and Evidence

Question 12 For each of the following scenarios, comment on the treatments and give evidence to support your views.

A 76-year-old man with Parkinson's disease

A 29-year-old woman with premenstrual syndrome (PMS)

A 74-year-old man with benign prostatic hypertrophy (BPH)

Paper 4

Question 1   You see a 31-year-old man who has a purulent urethral discharge. Outline your management.

Question 2   You are telephoned by the daughter of Mr Smith, an 81-year-old widower who lives alone. She lives in Canada and visits infrequently. She says that he is unsafe living alone and wants you to put him into a home. What issues does this raise?

Question 3 A 14-year-old boy comes to see you with his parents, He has just been discharged from hospital after having an epileptic seizure. What issues would you aim to cover and what would be your management aims?

Question 4   You practice in a busy urban practice with high deprivation scores. One of your partners announces at the practice meeting that he wants to become a trainer. What are the implications of his request?

Question 5   Discuss the usefulness of the following in the diagnosis and
management of eating disorders. Give evidence to support your
views:

Diagnostic tools
Cognitive behavioural therapy (CBT)
Drug therapy

Question 6   **What are the difficulties when dealing with patients who abuse opiate drugs?**

Question 7   **Outline ways in which practices can improve access for the disabled.**

Question 8   Mr Smith consults you with symptoms of atrial fibrillation. What evidence is there to help you decide on the value of the following aspects of care?

Control of rate
Reducing risk of thromboembolism
Control of rhythm

Question 9 Mr Jones, who has complained of impotence since being treated for a heart attack, asks for a prescription for sildenafil (Viagra), which you have not previously prescribed. You agree to look into it and come across an article entitled 'Systematic review of randomized controlled trials of sildenafil (Viagra) in the treatment of male erectile dysfunction' (with copyright permission from *British Journal of General Practice* 2001; 51: 1004–1011; reference material 4.1).

Comment on the selection process used

Comment on the studies identified

Comment on the endpoints used

Comment on the results in Fig.1 and their applicability to Mr Jones

Reference material 4.1a

Method

All published or unpublished randomised controlled trials comparing sildenafil with a placebo or alternative therapies were sought. Published studies were sought by computerised searches of electronic databases (MedLine, EMBASE, PsychLIT, Cochrane Library, National Research Register, Pharmline, PreMedline) in June 1999, using the keywords 'sildenafil' and 'Viagra'. There were no language restrictions. Internet search engines were used with the terms 'sildenafil' and 'Viagra'. In addition, a hand search was done of the *British Medical Journal, The Lancet, Journal of the American Medical Association, New England Journal of Medicine, British Journal of General Practice, Drug, Inpharma* and *Scrip* up to January 1999. A key source of information was the Food and Drug Administration (FDA) Center for Drug Evaluation and Research Joint Clinical Review for NDA-20-895 Viagra® (Sildenafil). Pfizer Ltd was contacted, as were experts in the field. References of all relevant studies were searched for further trial citations. The Science Citation Index was searched using all the studies identified.

An assessment of quality of all identified studies and data extraction was undertaken independently by two researchers, and they looked at concealment of allocation, blinding, losses to follow-up and intention-to-treat analysis. Discrepancies were resolved by discussion. Sildenafil is a new drug and all trials prior to its being licensed were sponsored by the drug company Pfizer. Where trials were only available in abstract form, further information was requested from Pfizer.

Primary outcome was defined as sexual function, as measured by questions 3 and 4 (03 and 04) of the International Index of Erectile Function (IIEF). The IIEF is a questionnaire consisting of 15 items designed to measure sexual and erectile function (Box 1). It was specifically developed and validated to evaluate sildenafil. Question 3 asks 'Over the past four weeks, when you have attempted sexual intercourse how often were you able to penetrate (enter) your partner?' Question 4 asks 'Over the past four weeks, during sexual intercourse, how often were you able to maintain your erection after you have penetrated (entered) your partner?' Responses are rated on a five-point ordinal scale. Zero is scored when responders did not attempt intercourse.

Secondary outcomes were composed of other questions on the IIEF, the global efficacy question 'Did treatment improve your erections?', measures of penile rigidity, an event log (of attempted and successful intercourse), and a partner questionnaire.

Results were combined in a meta-analysis where appropriate, using RevMan version 3.

Trials Identified

[Table 1 (opposite)]

Table 1 All Phase II and Phase III trials identified

Study ID, location, and date	Source of information	Study design	Duration	n	Treatment	Outcomes measured	Cause of ED in trial participants	Patient characteristics
Phase II trials to evaluate penile rigidity								
105 USA Multi-centre 1996	FDA NUA-20-895[6]	4-period crossover 1-week washout	1 dose	54 54 53 53	Placebo Sildenafil 25 mg Sildenafil 50 mg Sildenafil 100 mg	Duration of ⩾60% rigidity Duration of ⩾80% rigidity	Broad aetiology (excluding spinal cord injury)	Mean age between 51–55 Mean duration of ED not reported
350 UK Single-centre 1993	FDA NDA-20-895[6]	2-period crossover 1-week washout	7 days	16 16	Placebo Sildenafil 25 mg	Duration of >60% rigidity Duration of >80% rigidity Event log	No established organic cause	Mean age not reported Mean duration of ED not reported
351 (Part 1) UK Single-centre 1994	FDA NDA-20-895[6] Boolell et al 1996[9]	4-period crossover ⩾3-day washout	1 dose	12 12 12 12	Placebo Sildenafil 10 mg Sildenafil 25 mg Sildenafil 50 mg	Duration of >60% rigidity Duration of >80% rigidity	No established organic cause	Mean age = 48 (range = 36–63) Mean duration of ED = 3.4 years
357 (Part 1) UK Multi-centre 1994/95	FDA NDA-20-895[6] Price DE et al 1998[21]	3-period crossover 3–10 day washout	1 dose	21 21 21	Placebo Sildenafil 25 mg Sildenafil 50 mg	Duration of >60% rigidity Duration of >80% rigidity	Diabetes	Mean age = 50 (range = 29–66) Mean duration of ED = 3 years (range = 1–14) Diabetes > 5 years
358 (Part 1) UK Multi-centre 1995/96	FDA NDA-20-895[6] Maytom MC et al 1999[22]	2-period crossover 3–7 day washout	1 dose	27 27	Placebo Sildenafil 50 mg	Duration of >60% rigidity	Spinal cord injury (cord level range T6–L4/5)	Mean age = 33 (range = 21–49) Mean duration of ED = 6 years. Erectile response to vibrator
360 UK Single-centre 1995/96	Eardley et al 1997[27] (abstract) Boolell et al 1996[28] (abstract)	2-period crossover 1-week washout	1 dose	17 17	Placebo Sildenafil 50 mg	Duration of >60 % rigidity	No established organic cause	Mean age = 52 (range = 36–70) Median duration of ED = 1.5 years
369 UK Single-centre 1996	FDA NDA-20-895[7]	4-period crossover ⩾1-week washout	1 dose	16 16 16 16	Placebo Sildenafil 100 mg Placebo Sildenafil 100 mg	Duration of >60% rigidity 4 hours after dose Duration of >60% rigidity 2 hours after dose	No established organic cause	Mean age = 55 years Mean duration of ED = 4.5 years
166–301 1995	Pfizer study report	3-period crossover ⩾3-day washout	1 dose	10 10	Placebo Sildenafil 50 mg	Duration of >60% rigidity	No established organic cause	Age range = 32–69 ED for 3 months or more
Phase II and III trials with clinical outcomes								
101 USA Multi-centre 1995/96	FDA NDA-20-895[7] Leu et al 1997[15] (abstract)	Fixed dose Parallel group 2–4 week treatment-free run in	24 weeks	83 86 82 83 82	Placebo Sildenafil 5 mg Sildenafil 25 mg Sildenafil 50 mg Sildenafil 100 mg	Sexual function questionnaire Event log Partner questionnaire	Broad aetiology (excluding spinal cord injury)	Mean age = 57.6 years Mean duration of ED = 4.6 years

Table 1 (continued)

Study ID, location and date	Source of information	Study design.	Duration	n	Treatment	Outcomes measured	Cause of ED in trial participants	Patient characteristics
102 USA Multi-centre 1995/96	FDA NDA-20-895[7] Goldstein et al 1998[8] Pfizer study report	Fixed dose Parallel group 4-week treatment-free run in	24 weeks	216 102 107 107	Placebo Sildenafil 25 mg Sildenafil 50 mg Sildenafil 100 mg	IIEF Global efficacy question Quality of life questionnaire Partner questionnaire Pharmacokinetic data	Broad aetiology (excluding spinal cord injury)	Mean age = 57.6 years Mean duration of ED = 3.2 years
103 USA Multi-centre 1996	FDA NDA-20-895[7] Goldstein et al 1998[8] Pfizer study report	Variable dose Parallel group 4-week treatment-free run in	12 weeks	166 163	Placebo Sildenafil 25–100 mg	IIEF Global efficacy question Quality of life questionnaire Partner questionnaire Pharmacokinetic data	Broad aetiology (excluding spinal cord injury)	Mean age = 59.5 years Mean duration of ED = 4.8 years
104 USA Multi-centre 1996	FDA NDA-20-895[7] Rendell et al 1999[16] Pfizer study report	Variable dose Parallel group 4-week treatment free run in	12 weeks	132 136	Placebo Sildenafil 50–100 mg	IIEF Global efficacy question Quality of life questionnaire Partner questionnaire Pharmacokinetic data	Diabetes	Mean age = 57 years Mean duration of ED = 5.6 years Mean duration of diabetes = 12.1 years 18.7% type 1, 81.3% type 2 diabetes
106 Canada Multi-centre 1996/97	FDA NDA-20-895[7] Pfizer study report	Fixed dose Parallel group 4-week treatment-free run in	12 weeks	122 127 124 124	Placebo Sildenafil 50 mg Sildenafil 100 mg Sildenafil 200 mg	IIEF Global efficacy question Quality of life questionnaire Partner questionnaire Pharmacokinetic data	Broad aetiology (excluding spinal cord injury)	Mean age = 58 years Mean duration of ED = 5.4 years
351 (Part 11) UK Single centre 1994	FDA NDA-20-895[7] Boolell et al 1996[9]	2-period crossover 7-day washout	7 days	12 12	Placebo Sildenafil 25 mg	Patient diary	No established organic cause	Mean age 48 = (range = 36-63) Mean duration of ED = 3.4 years
353 Europe Multi-centre 1994/95	FDA NDA-20-895[7] Dinsmore et al 1996[17] (abstract)	Fixed dose Parallel group 2-week treatment-free run in	4 weeks	95 90 85 81	Placebo Sildenafil 10 mg Sildenafil 25 mg Sildenafil 50 mg	Sexual function questionnaire Global efficacy question Event log	No established organic cause	Mean age = 53 years Mean duration of ED = 4.5 years
355 UK Multi-centre 1994/95	FDA NDA-20-895[7] Eardley et al 1996[18] (abstract)	Variable dose crossover 3-week treatment-free run in	4 weeks X 2 no washout	43 44	Placebo Sildenafil 25–75 mg	Global efficacy question Event log	No established organic cause	Mean age = 53 years Mean duration of ED = 3 years

Study / Region / Year	Reference	Design	Duration	n	Treatment	Assessment measures	Aetiology	Demographics
356 Europe Multi-centre 1994/95	FDA NDA-20-895[7] Bailey et al 1997[19] (abstract) Virag et al 1996[20] (abstract)	Variable dose Parallel group	8 weeks	106 99	Placebo Sildenafil 10-100 mg	Sexual function questionnaire Global efficacy question Event log	Broad aetiology	Mean age = 54 years Mean duration of ED = 4.9 years
357 (Part II) UK Multi-centre 1994/95	FDA NDA-20-895[7] Price et al 1998[21]	3-period crossover 3-10 day washout	10 days	21 21 21	Placebo Sildenafil 25 mg Sildenafil 50 mg	Global efficacy question Event log	Diabetes	Mean age = 50 (range = 29-66) Mean duration of ED = 3 years (range = 1-14), Diabetes > 5 years
358 (Part II) UK Multi-centre 1995/96	FDA NDA-20-895[7] Maytom MC et al 1999[22]	Fixed dose Parallel group	4 weeks	14 12	Placebo Sildenafil 50 mg	Sexual function questionnaire Global efficacy question Event log Partner questionnaire	Spinal cord injury (cord level range T6-L4/5)	Mean age = 33 (range 21-49) Mean duration of ED = 6 years. Erectile response to vibrator
359 UK Multi-centre 1995/96	FDA NDA20-895 7 Abel et al 1997[12] (abstract) Pfizer study report	Variable dose Parallel group 2-4 treatment-free run in period	12 weeks	54 57	Placebo Sildenafil 25-100 mg	IIEF Global efficacy question Event log	Broad aetiology	Mean age = 56 years Mean duration of ED = 4.5 years
361 Australia Multi-centre 1996	FDA NDA-20-895[7] Pfizer study report	Fixed dose Parallel group 2-week treatment-free run in	12 weeks	59 62 66 67	Placebo Sildenafil 50 mg Sildenafil 100 mg Sildenafil 200 mg	IIEF Global efficacy question Event log	Organic aetiology (excluding spinal cord injury)	Mean age = 57 years Mean duration of ED = 5.2 years
363 Europe Multi-centre 1995196	FDA NDA-20-895[7] Cuzin et al 1997[13] (abstract) Pfizer study report	Variable dose Parallel group 4-week treatment-free run in	26 weeks	156 159	Placebo Sildenafil 25-100 mg	IIEF Global efficacy question Event log Quality of life questionnaire Partner questionnaire	Broad aetiology	Mean age = 54.5 years Mean duration = 4.8 years
364 Europe Multi-centre 1996	FDA NDA-20-895[7] Pfizer study report	Fixed dose Parallel group 4-week treatment-free run in	12 weeks	127 128 132 127	Placebo Sildenafil 25 mg Sildenafil 50 mg Sildenafil 100 mg	IIEF Global efficacy question Event log Quality of life questionnaire Partner questionnaire Pharmacokinetic data	Broad aetiology	Mean age = 55.8 years Duration of ED = 4.8 years
367 Europe & Australia Multi-centre 1996/97	FDA NDA-20-895[7] Giuliano et al 1999[4]	Variable dose crossover 4-week treatment-free run in	6 weeks X 2 separated by a 2-week washout	178 178	Placebo Sildenafil 25-100 mg	IIEF Global efficacy question Event log Quality of life questionnaire Partner questionnaire	Spinal cord injury	Mean age = 38 years Mean duration of ED = 11 years

Results Figure 1

Comparison: 05 Sildenafil compared with placebo
Outcome: 01 Global Efficacy Question

Study	Experiment n/N	Control n/N	Risk difference (95% CI Random)	Weight %	Risk difference (95% CI Random)
101	202/310	22/74		6.6	0.354 (0.237–0.471)
102	209/293	53/194		8.0	0.440 (0.359–0.521)
103	101/136	23/141		7.5	0.580 (0.484–0.675)
104	74/131	13/127		7.3	0.463 (0.363–0.562)
106	262/338	27/108		7.5	0.525 (0.432–0.618)
351	10/12	2/12		2.4	0.667 (0.368–0.965)
353	186/242	35/91		6.8	0.384 (0.217–0.497)
355	36/44	10/44		4.9	0.591 (0.423–0.759)
356	81/99	28/106		6.8	0.554 (0.441–0.667)
357	11/21	2/21		3.1	0.429 (0.181–0.676)
358	18/27	2/27		4.0	0.593 (0.389–0.796)
359	42/52	7/39		5.1	0.628 (0.467–0.789)
361	128/167	6/47		6.7	0.639 (0.524–0.754)
363	117/142	29/121		7.3	0.584 (0.486–0.683)
364	276/359	27/114		7.7	0.532 (0.443–0.621)
367	142/175	21/174		8.2	0.691 (0.615–0.766)
Total (95% CI)	1895/2548	307/1440		100.0	0.537 (0.484–0.589)

$\chi^2 = 49.17$ (df = 15); $Z = 19.88$

−1   0   1

Favours control   Favours treatment

Figure 1 Meta-analysis of results for global efficacy question

Question 10 Statins: a panacea for all ills? Comment, with reference to current evidence.

Question 11 Your practice is looking at designing a protocol for the management of blood pressure in the nurse-led diabetic clinic. You wish the process to be evidence-based. See reference material 4.2a, an extract from the paper 'Tight blood pressure control and risk of macrovascular and microvascular complications in type 2 diabetes:UK PDS 38' (with copyright permission from *British Medical Journal* 1998; 317: 703–13)

Comment on the strengths and weaknesses of the methodology

Comment on the results shown in Fig. 4 (reference material 4.2b)

Comment on the overall validity of the results

Comment on the generalisability of the results to general practice

Reference Material 4.2a

We studied hypertensive patients with type 2 diabetes who had been recruited to the UK prospective diabetes study. General practitioners were asked to refer patients aged 25–65 with newly diagnosed diabetes to 23 participating centres. A total of 5102 were recruited as they met the study's entry criterion (fasting plasma glucose concentration >6 mmol/l on two mornings), were willing to join, and did not meet the exclusion criteria for the study. Exclusion criteria were ketonuria >3 mmol/l; a history of myocardial infarction in the previous year; current angina or heart failure; more than one major vascular episode; serum creatinine concentration >175 μmol/l; retinopathy requiring laser treatment; malignant hypertension; an uncorrected endocrine abnormality; an occupation which would preclude insulin treatment (such as heavy goods vehicle driver); a severe concurrent illness likely to limit life or require extensive systemic treatment; or inadequate understanding or unwillingness to enter the study. The patients were treated by diet alone for 3 months. Patients who remained hyperglycaemic (fasting plasma glucose 6.1–15.0 mmol/l) without diabetic symptoms were randomly allocated conventional blood glucose control, primarily by diet, or intensive control (aiming for a fasting plasma glucose concentration <6.0 mmol/l) with additional sulphonylurea, insulin, or metformin treatment. Details of the protocol are published.

   Of the 4297 patients recruited to the 20 centres participating in the hypertension in diabetes study, 243 had either died or were lost to follow up before the start of the hypertension study in 1987. Of the remaining 4054 patients, 1544 (38%) had hypertension, defined in 727 patients as a systolic blood pressure ≥160 mm Hg and/or a diastolic blood pressure ≥90 mm Hg or in 421 patients receiving antihypertensive treatment as a systolic pressure of ≥150 mm Hg and/or a diastolic blood pressure ≥85 Hg. Patients were enrolled on the basis of the mean of three blood pressure measurements taken at consecutive clinic visits. The exclusion criteria were a clinical requirement for strict blood pressure control (previous stroke, accelerated hypertension, cardiac failure, or renal failure) or β blockade (myocardial infarction in the previous year or current angina); severe vascular disease (more than one major vascular episode); a severe concurrent illness or contraindications to β blockers (asthma, intermittent claudication, foot ulcers, or amputations); pregnancy; or unwillingness to join the study. Of the 1544 hypertensive patients, 252 were excluded and 144 patients did not enter the study. A total of 1148 patients (637 men (55%) with a mean age of 56.4 (SD 8.1) years entered the hypertension in diabetes study between 1987 and 1991. Table 1 shows their characteristics at randomisation to blood pressure control policy.

Treatment protocol

Randomisation stratified for those with or without previous treatment for hypertension was performed by the coordinating centre. In all 758 patients were allocated tight control of blood pressure, aiming for a blood pressure <150/ 85 mm Hg (400 patients were given an angiotensin converting enzyme inhibitor (captopril) and 358 a β blocker (atenolol) as the main treatment); 390 patients were allocated a less tight control of blood pressure, aiming for a blood pressure <180/105 mm Hg but avoiding treatment with angiotensin converting enzyme inhibitors or β blockers. Sealed opaque envelopes were used and checked as described for the UK prospective diabetes study. The original blood pressure target of 200/105mm Hg in the group assigned to less tight control was reduced in 1992 by the steering committee of the hypertension in diabetes study after publication of the results of studies in elderly, non-diabetic subjects during 1991–2. Randomisation produced balanced numbers of patients allocated to the various glucose and blood pressure treatment combinations for the UK prospective diabetes study and hypertension in diabetes study.

Captopril was usually started at a dose of 25 mg twice daily, increasing to 50mg twice daily, and atenolol at a daily dose of 50 mg, increasing to 100 mg if required. Other agents were added if the control criteria were not met in the group assigned to tight control despite maximum allocated treatment or in the group assigned to less tight control without drug treatment. The suggested sequence was frusemide 20 mg daily (maximum 40 mg twice daily), slow release nifedipine 10mg (maximum 40 mg) twice daily, methyldopa 250 mg (maximum 500 mg) twice daily, and prazosin 1 mg (maximum 5 mg) thrice daily.

Clinic visits

Patients visited study clinics every 3–4 months. At each visit plasma glucose concentration, blood pressure, and body weight were measured, and treatments to control blood pressure and blood glucose concentration were noted and adjusted if target values were not met. If treatments and target blood pressures were not in accord with the protocol, the coordinating centre sent letters about affected patients to the clinical centres requesting appropriate action. A central record of all apparent protocol deviations was maintained. Symptoms including any drug side effects and clinical events were noted. Physicians recorded hypoglycaemic episodes as minor if the patient was able to treat the symptoms unaided and as major if third party or medical intervention was necessary.

Blood pressure measurements

Blood pressure (diastolic phase 5) while the patient was sitting and had rested for at least five minutes was measured by a trained nurse with a Copal UA-251 or a Takeda UA-751 electronic auscultatory blood pressure reading machine (Andrew Stephens, Brighouse, West Yorkshire) or with a Hawksley random zero sphygmomanometer (Hawksley, Lancing, Sussex) in patients with atrial fibrillation. The first reading was discarded and the mean of the next three consecutive readings with a coefficient of variation below 15% was used in the study, with additional readings if required. Monthly quality assurance measurements have shown the mean difference between Takeda and Hawksley machines to be 1 (4) mm Hg or less.

Clinical examination

At entry to the UK prospective diabetes study and subsequently every three years all patients had a clinical examination which included retinal colour photography, ophthalmoscopy, measurement of visual acuity, assessment of peripheral and autonomic neuropathy, chest radiography, electrocardiography, and measurement of brachial and posterior tibial blood pressure using Doppler techniques. Annual direct ophthalmoscopy was also carried out. Every year a fasting blood sample was taken to measure glycated haemoglobin (haemoglobin A_{1c}), plasma creatinine concentration, and concentrations of urea, immunoreactive insulin, and insulin antibodies; random urine samples were taken for measurement of albumin concentration.

Visual acuity was measured with Snellen charts until 1989, after which ETDRS (early treatment of diabetic retinopathy study) charts were used to assess best corrected vision, with current refraction or through a pinhole. Retinal colour photographs of four standard 30° fields per eye (nasal, disc, macula, and temporal to macular fields) were taken plus stereophotographs of the macula. Repeat photography was arranged if the quality of the photograph was unsatisfactory. Retinal photographs were assessed at a central grading centre by two independent assessors for the presence or absence of diabetic retinopathy. Any fields with retinopathy were graded by two further senior independent assessors using a modified ETDRS final scale. Neuropathy was assessed clinically by knee and ankle reflexes, and by biothesiometer (Biomedical Instruments, Newbury, Ohio) readings taken from the lateral malleoli and the end of the big toe. A 12 lead electrocardiogram was recorded and given a Minnesota code, and a chest x ray film was taken for measurement of cardiac diameter.

Biochemistry

Biochemical methods have been reported previously. Urinary albumin concentration was measured by an immunoturbidimetric method with a normal reference range of 1.4 mg/l to 36.5 mg/l. Microalbuminuria has been defined as a urinary albumin concentration of $\geqslant 50$ mg/l and clinical grade proteinuria as a urinary albumin concentration of $\geqslant 300$ mg/l.

Clinical end points

Twenty one clinical end points were predefined in the study protocol. All available clinical information was gathered for possible end points – for example, copies of admission notes, operation records, death certificates, and necropsy reports. Copies of these, without reference to the patient's allocated or actual treatment, were formally presented to two independent physicians who allocated an appropriate code from the ninth revision of the international classification of diseases (ICD-9) if the criteria for any particular clinical end point had been met. Any disagreement between the two assessors was discussed and the evidence reviewed. If agreement was not possible the information was submitted to a panel of two further independent assessors for final arbitration. The closing date for the study was 30 September 1997.

End points were aggregated for the main analyses. The three predefined primary outcome analyses were the time to the occurrence of (a) a first clinical end point related to diabetes (sudden death, death from hyperglycaemia or hypoglycaemia, fatal or non-fatal myocardial infarction, angina, heart failure, stroke, renal failure, amputation (of at least one digit), vitreous haemorrhage, retinal photocoagulation, blindness in one eye or cataract extraction); (b) death related to diabetes (death due to myocardial infarction, sudden death, stroke, peripheral vascular disease, renal disease, hyperglycaemia or hypoglycaemia); (c) death from all causes.

Secondary outcome analyses of four additional aggregates of clinical end points were used to assess the effect of treatments on different types of vascular disease. These were myocardial infarction (fatal or non-fatal myocardial infarction or sudden death), stroke (fatal or non-fatal stroke), amputation or death from peripheral vascular disease, and microvascular complications (retinopathy requiring photocoagulation, vitreous haemorrhage, and fatal or non-fatal renal failure).

Since a patient could in sequence have different end points, he or she could be included in more than one end point category.

Surrogate end points – Details of subclinical, surrogate variables have been published.

Statistical analysis

Analysis was on an intention to treat basis, comparing patients allocated to tight and less tight blood pressure control. Patients allocated to tight control with angiotensin converting enzyme inhibitors or β blockers were pooled in this paper for analysis. They are compared in the accompanying paper. Life table analyses were performed with log rank tests, and hazard ratios were obtained from Cox's proportional hazards models and used to estimate relative risks. Survival function estimates were calculated using the product limit (Kaplan–Meier) method. In the text relative risks are quoted as risk reductions and significance tests were two sided. For aggregate end points 95% confidence intervals are quoted, whereas for single end points 99% confidence intervals are quoted to allow for potential type 1 errors. Similarly, 99% confidence intervals were used to assess surrogate end points that were measured at triennial visits. Mean (SD), geometric mean (1SD interval), or median (interquartile range) values are quoted for the biometric and biochemical variables, with values from Wilcoxon, t, or χ^2 tests for comparisons. Risk reductions for surrogate end points were derived from frequency tables. The overall values for blood pressure during a period were assessed for each patient as the mean during that period and for each allocation as the mean of patients with data in the allocation. Control of blood pressure was assessed in patients allocated to the two groups who had data at nine years of follow up.

Hypoglycaemia was determined from the number of patients allocated to a treatment and continuing with it who had one or more minor or major hypoglycaemic episodes each year. Urinary albumin concentration was measured in mg/l. Change in diabetic retinopathy was defined as a change of two steps (one step in both eyes or two or more steps in one eye) with a scale from the worse eye to the better eye that included retinal photocoagulation or vitreous haemorrhage as the most serious grade. Visual loss was defined as the best vision in either eye, deteriorating by three lines on an ETDRS chart. Both the UK prospective diabetes study and hypertension in diabetes study received ethical approval from the appropriate committee in each centre and conformed with the guidelines of the Declarations of Helsinki (1975 and 1983). All patients gave informed consent.

Reference material 4.2b

Clinical end point	Patients with aggregate end points			Absolute risk (events per 1000 patient years)			Relative risk for tight control (95% CI)
	Tight control (n = 758)	Less tight control (n = 390)	Tight control	Less tight control	p value		
Any diabetes related end point	259	170	50. 9	67.4	0.0046	0.76 (0.62 to 0.92)
Deaths related to diabetes	82	62	13.7	20.3	0.019	0.68 (0.49 to 0.94)
All cause mortality	134	83	22.4	27.2	0.17	0.82 (0.63 to 1.08)
Myocardial infarction	107	69	18.6	23.5	0.13	0.79 (0.59 to 1.07)
Stroke	38	34	6.5	11.6	0.013	0.56 (0.35 to 0.89)
Peripheral vascular disease	8	8	1.4	2.7	0.17	0.51 (0.19 to 1.37)
Microvascular disease	68	54	12.0	19.2	0.0092	0.63 (0.44 to 0.89)

Favours tight control — Favours less tight control (scale 0.1 to 10)

Figure 4 Numbers of patients who attained one or more clinical end points in aggregates representing specific types of clinical complications, with relative risks comparing tight control of blood pressure with less tight control

Question 12   Your practice is attempting to shorten access times to comply with government targets. One of the areas you decide to concentrate on is frequent attenders. See reference material 4.3a, an extract from 'Psychosocial, lifestyle, and health status variables in predicting high attendance among adults' (with copyright permission from *British Journal of General Practice* 2001; 51: 987–994)

Comment on the strengths and weaknesses of the methodology

Comment on the results given in Table 2 and Table 4 of reference material 4.3b

Suggest possible interventions based on these results

Reference Material 4.3a

Method

Six general practices within a 30-mile radius of the administrative centre were chosen to give a range of sociodemographic and practice characteristics. A sample of 4000 households was randomly chosen, using equal numbers from the age–sex register of each practice. Patients from nursing homes and those aged over 80 years old were excluded owing to difficulty in completing the questionnaire. Patients were sent a letter explaining the project, the questionnaire, and one of three types of information leaflet/booklet. The cohort was followed to assess the effectiveness of the leaflets (these results will be reported elsewhere). One adult per household was sampled to avoid contamination of groups. Where the random choice of participant from the age–sex register was a child (aged under 16 years, $n = 487$) an adult was asked to fill in a questionnaire for themselves, in addition to one for the child: this paper reports the adults' data. A second and third mailing were sent to patients who had not responded to the first questionnaire.

Questionnaire

Existing measures. We included items from previous studies, questions about lifestyle, and attitudes.

New measures. To limit type I error, where variables potentially addressed similar domains, exploratory factor analysis with varimax rotation was performed to identify a smaller number of 'latent' variables. Scales were developed based on a simple sum of the items which loaded strongly for each factor. 'New' measures included:

Health status (modified COOP WONCA chart questions). The chart component was omitted for ease of printing and scanning, leaving the wording unchanged. Factor analysis suggested a two-factor solution:

(a) 'physical health' – physical activity (rotated factor loading 0.50), bodily discomfort/pain (0.52), ability to work (0.65), and overall condition (0.50). A higher score represents poorer 'physical health' status. Cronbach's cx for the scale was 0.72, i.e. in the optimum range.

(b) 'social/emotional health' – emotional problems (0.69), social activities (0.53), quality of life (0.71), and overall functioning (0.62) (cx = 0.81). Questions about social support and change in condition did not load strongly onto either 'physical' or 'emotional' factors.

The validity of the word format was compared with the original chart version sent one month later in 32 consecutive responders (Spearman's p = 0.80 for 'physical'; p = 0.79 for 'social/emotional').

Willingness to tolerate symptoms. Thirteen questions documented the number of days that people would wait before seeing the doctor for clinical scenarios (1 = less than one day; 2 = one to two days; 3 = three to seven days; 4 = eight to 14 days; 5 = over 14 days; 6 = would not contact). Factor analysis suggested a one-factor solution. Seven questions 'loaded' strongly: headache (0.62), consti-pation (0.67), diarrhoea and vomiting (0.62), indigestion and heartburn (0.66), cold and runny nose (0.64), 'flu with fever (0.66), sore throat and fever (0.71) (a = **0.8322**). Test–retest reliability of the scale after one month in 32 people was acceptable (p = 0.48).

'Personality'. Questions were based on Kokko's descriptions of personality types in high attenders (1 = 'very strongly agree', through to 7 = very strongly dis-agree'). Factor analysis suggested a three-factor solution.

(a) Factor 1 ('demedicalise') – 'the importance of the doctor making sure there is nothing seriously wrong' (0.56), 'the doctor checking things out quickly when unwell' (0.60), 'liking to find out as much as possible when unwell' (0.69), 'liking referral to specialist when possible' (0.73), 'liking tests when unwell' (0.75), 'wanting to know about side-effects' (0.55), and 'wanting the doctor to do something about it when unwell' (0.59) (a = 0.83).

(b) Factor 2 ('positive and interested') this 'loaded' questions about: 'changing health being outside my control' (0.56), 'my problems are more serious than the doctor thinks' (0.57), 'being worried when the doctor goes into details' (0.57), and 'wanting to just have the treatment without the doctor going into reasons' (0.62) (c~ = 0.69).

(c) Factor 3 ('medophile') this 'loaded' questions about: 'dislike of taking medi-cines and remedies' (0.51) 'and most illnesses get better without medicines' (0.50) (a = 0.58, owing to being only two items).

The question scoring meant that higher scores for the three factors reflected patients who disliked the medical process, were positive and interested in health, and positive about medicines, respectively. Other questions derived from Kokko's descriptions did not load onto the above factors – including 'repeated visits are normally needed to get the right treatment'.

Self-reported attendance
We were interested in those consulting the doctor or nurse more frequently than the average, i.e. five or more attendances a year (the top 25%, accounting *for* the majority [60%] of consultations). We assessed test–retest reliability of the question about self-reported attendance in the first 32 responders after one month. We also compared self-reported attendance for attendance documented in the notes in 270 consecutive responders.

Sample size (/3 = 0.2, a = 0.05 using the EPI INFO software)
To detect risk factors with an odds ratio of 2 for high attendance, where the prevalence of higher attendance in patients with risk factors ranges from 10% to 90% and the prevalence of exposure ranges from 20% to 80%, 2202 responders were required (or 3146 allowing for 30% non-response).

Analysis

Data were scanned using Formic 3 software and analysis performed using SPSS and Stata for Windows software. Variables significantly associated with attendance (five or more per year) were entered in logistic regression models by forward selection, and retained if they remained significant (using the likelihood ratio test) and no evidence of significant multi-collinearity. To allow the reader to better assess the risk' associated with significant continuous variables (e.g. somatic symptom inventory, health anxiety) they were converted to ordinal variables: cut-offs were determined by the shape of the relationship with outcome rather than using pre-determined arbitrary cut-offs. The large sample allowed us to choose a 1% level of significance to limit type I error: a 1% level rather than the more conservative Bonferroni correction was chosen owing to close interrelation of many of the variables and collinearity of the hypotheses being tested. The adequacy of the model in predicting outcome was assessed by calculating the area under the receiver operator characteristic CR00) curve.

Reference material 4.3b

[Tables 2 and 4]

Table 2 Sociodemographic, life events and practice variables associated with self-reported higher attendance at GP surgery (five or more times in past 12 months)

Variable	High attender (%)	Not a high attender (%)	Crude odds ratio (95% CI)	Adjusted odds ratio (95% CI)[a]	Likelihood ratio[b] χ^2 (P-value)
Sociodemographic					
Age (years)					
20	24/625 (4)	121/1901 (6)	1	1	6.5 (P = 0.090)
20–39	196/625 (31)	657/1901 (35)	1.50 (0.94–2.40)	1.77 (0.90–3.46)	
40–64	263/625 (42)	869/1901 (46)	1.53 (0.96–2.41)	1.28 (0.66–2.51)	
>64	142/625 (23)	254/1901 (13)	2.82 (1.74–4.57)	1.50 (0.72–3.11)	
Sex (female)	423/622 (68)	1083/1898 (57)	1.60 (1.32–1.94)	1.44 (1.11–1.87)	7.5 (P = 0.006)
No qualifications	257/593 (43)	479/1814 (26)	2.13 (1.76–2.59)	1.61 (1.25–2.07)	13.6 (P < 0.001)
Children at home	354/623 (57)	907/1869 (49)	1.40 (1.16–1.68)	1.07 (0.84–1.37)	0.3 (P = 0.586)
Ethnicity (non–white)	12/623 (2)	24/1887 (1)	1.52 (0.76–3.07)	1.42 (0.56–3.56)	0.5 (P = 0.464)
Marital status					
Single	92/628 (15)	317/1904 (17)	1	1	1.1 (P = 0.570)
Married	427/628 (68)	1333/1904 (70)	1.10 (0.85–1.43)	0.83 (0.58–1.18)	
Separated/widowed/divorced	109/628 (17)	254/1904 (13)	1.48 (1.07–2.04)	0.83 (0.53–1.30)	
Council house tenant	134/603 (22)	230/1859 (12)	2.02 (1.60–2.56)	1.32 (0.93–1.85)	2.4 (P = 0.118)
Occupation					
Paid employment	311/601 (52)	1316/1865 (71)	1	1	6.7 (P = 0.145)
Homemaker	62/601 (10)	174/1865 (9)	1.51 (1.10–2.07)	0.86 (0.56–1.31)	
Retired	170/601 (28)	298/1865 (16)	2.41 (1.93–3.02)	1.32 (0.95–1.82)	
Disabled	42/601 (7)	22/1865 (1)	8.08 (4.75–13.73)	1.83 (0.86–3.91)	
Unemployed	16/601 (3)	45/1865 (2)	1.50 (0.84–2.70)	1.58 (0.79–3.18)	
Life events					
0	233/630 (37)	836/1913 (44)	1	1	1.1 (P = 0.773)
1	224/630 (36)	617/1913 (32)	1.30 (1.05–1.61)	1.13 (0.85–1.49)	
2	110/630 (17)	302/1913 (16)	1.31 (1.01–1.70)	1.05 (0.74–1.48)	
3+	63/630 (10)	158/1913 (8)	1.43 (1.03–1.98)	1.20 (0.79–1.82)	
Practice					
1 U; A; F; C; DI	105/630 (17)	279/1913 (15)	1	1	8.3 (P = 0.140)
2 U; T; DI	117/630 (19)	281/1913 (15)	1.11 (0.81–1.51)	0.92 (0.60–1.39)	
3 U; DI	101/630 (16)	282/1913 (15)	0.95 (0.69–1.31)	0.80 (0.52–1.23)	
4 U; F; C; 1; T	110/630 (17)	330/1913 (17)	0.89 (0.65–1.21)	0.99 (0.65–1.50)	
5 U; 1	103/630 (16)	335/1913 (18)	0.82 (0.60–1.12)	0.78 (0.51–1.18)	
6 U/R; 1, C; F; M	94/630 (15)	406/1913 (21)	0.62 (0.45–0.84)	0.61 (0.40–0.92)	

[a] Adjusted for other variables that were significantly associated with attendance. [b] Likelihood ratio test. U predominantly urban; U/R = urban rural mixed;
T = teaching; A = academic (linked to university department; F = fundholding; I = inner city; DI = deprived inner city; M = market town

Table 4 Somatic symptoms and health perception, attitude to doctors, and lifestyle variables that were significantly associated with self-reported higher attendance at the GP surgery (five or more times in past 12 months)

Variable	High attender %	Not a high attender %	Crude odds ratio (95% CI)	Adjusted odds ratio (95% CI)[a]	Likelihood ratio[b] χ^2 (P-value)
Symptom and health perception					
Medically unexplained symptoms					7.5 ($P = 0.006$)
0	113/630 (18)	653/1913 (34)	1	1	
1–2	172/630 (27)	626/1913 (33)	1.59 (1.22–2.06)	1.15 (0.81–1.62)	
3–5	181/630 (29)	430/1913 (22)	2.43 (1.87–3.17)	1.48 (1.04–2.09)	
6+	164/630 (26)	204/1913 (11)	4.65 (3.49–6.19)	1.62 (1.08–2.42)	
Health anxiety (Whitely Index)					10.9 ($P=0.001$)
0	33/630 (5)	160/1913 (8)	1	1	
1–5	478/630 (76)	1606/1913 (84)	1.44 (0.98–2.13)	1.22 (0.71–2.10)	
6–7	63/630 (10)	100/1913 (5)	3.05 (1.87–4.98)	1.77 (0.90–3.46)	
8+	56/630 (9)	47/1913 (2)	5.78 (3.37–9.91)	2.78 (1.31–5.89)	
Perceived health					15.4 ($P<0.001$)
Very good	85/610 (14)	590/1874 (31)	1	1	
Good	418/610 (69)	1204/1874 (64)	2.41 (1.87–3.10)	1.61 (1.12–2.33)	
Poor	107/610 (18)	80/1874 (4)	9.28 (6.42–13.42)	2.93 (1.71–5.03)	
Attitude to doctors					
Negative attitude (Negdoc scale)					22.1 ($P<0.001$)
<18	190/602 (32)	478/1844 (26)	1	1	
18–20	214/602 (36)	622/1844 (34)	0.87 (0.69–1.09)	0.83 (0.62–1.11)	
21+	198/602 (33)	744/1844 (40)	0.67 (0.53–0.84)	0.48 (0.36–0.66)	
Often need to reattend to get right treatment (% disagreeing)	331/609 (54)	1344/1874 (72)	0.47 (0.39–0.57)	0.61 (0.47–0.78)	14.6 ($P<0.001$)
Usually try chemist first (% agreeing)	352/612 (58)	1349/1884 (72)	0.54 (0.45–0.65)	0.61 (0.48–0.78)	15.2 ($P<0.001$)
Lifestyle					
Alcohol (units/day)					10.1 ($P=0.002$)
0	172/595 (29)	342/1822 (19)	1	1	
1	372/595 (63)	1200/1822 (66)	0.62 (0.50–0.77)	0.82 (0.61–1.09)	
2	36/595 (6)	176/1822 (10)	0.41 (0.27–0.61)	0.76 (0.46–1.27)	
3+	15/595 (3)	104/1822 (6)	0.29 (0.16–0.51)	0.25 (0.11–0.55)	
Sedentary (no brisk exercise)	253/610 (41)	632/1858 (34)	1.37 (1.14–1.66)	0.98 (0.76–1.27)	0.0 ($P=0.900$)
Smoking					0.2 ($P=0.892$)
Never	267/623 (43)	872/1884 (46)	1	1	
Ex-smoker	207/623 (33)	563/1884 (30)	1.20 (0.97–1.48)	0.93 (0.70–1.25)	
Current	149/623 (24)	449/1884 (24)	1.08 (0.86–1.36)	0.98 (0.72–1.34)	

[a]Adjusted for other variables which were significantly associated with attendance. [b]likelihood ratio test.

Paper 5

Question 1   A local headmaster with type 2 diabetes refuses to take medication, preferring homeopathic treatment. He refuses to attend the diabetic clinic. Bloods show a fasting blood sugar of 12, HbA1c 9.6. BP 184/102, BMI 36. How would you manage his care?

Question 2   Following an audit by the GP registrar it has been brought to your attention as trainer that one of the senior partners has been prescribing excessive amounts of benzodiazepines. What issues are raised by this?

Question 3   A 40-year-old civil engineer comes to you having recently been diagnosed with retinitis pigmentosa (autosomal dominant). He has two teenage daughters. What factors affect this consultation?

Question 4   Obesity is a common problem. Comment on the following, giving evidence to support your views:

The value of treating obesity
Drug treatment
Surgical treatment
Lifestyle measures

Question 5   How can burnout be avoided?

Question 6   How does the evidence contribute to the management of chest
infections in primary care? Comment under the following headings:

Diagnosis
Treatment

Question 7   As a result of an audit it has become clear that an excessive number of your patients fail to attend outpatient appointments after being referred by their GP. In a drive to improve access times you set up a working party to explore the causes of this. You wish the process to be evidence-based.

Outline how you would gather your evidence

Read reference material 5.1a, part of the paper from the *British Journal of General Practice* entitled 'Patient, hospital and general practitioner characteristics associated with non-attendance: a cohort study' (with copyright permission from BJGP 2002; 52 (477): 317–319).

Comment on the strengths and weaknesses of the methodology of the study as presented

Reference material 5.1a

Method

The study used a prospective cohort approach. It was run in parallel with a randomised controlled trial of an intervention aimed to reduce non-attendance. Twenty-six GPs from 13 practices in Exeter, UK, enrolled all new referrals between January and May 1997 into the study.

The patients' age, sex, and referral specialty (surgery; obstetrics and gynaecology; medicine; orthopaedics; ophthalmology; ear, nose and throat or oral surgery; dermatology; psychiatry; or other) were extracted from the referral letter. The Jarman score, as a proxy measure of socioeconomic status, was calculated from the postcode. The interval between referral and appointment was calculated from the referral and reply letters. GP details were obtained from the Health Authority. Referral rates were calculated from the number of referrals made during the study and the list size calculated from practice details.

Attendance data were obtained from routine hospital datasets, crosschecked by examination of the GP records. Cancellations were considered as attendances for analysis. Attendance rates between specialties were compared using a χ^2 test. All variables (sex, age, Jarman score, interval to appointment, specialty, fundholding status, referral rate, possession of Membership of the Royal College of General Practitioners, and year of qualification of GP) were entered into a univariable analysis. Logistic regression was performed using non-attendance versus cancellation or attendance as the outcome measure. Those variables with a probability of the null hypothesis of less than 0.2 were entered into a multivariable analysis.

Question 8   Extracts from the results section of the paper referred to in the preceding question are given in reference material 5.2a. With copyright permission from British Journal of General Practice.

What do you conclude from the results presented?

What other factors may explain the results seen?

Reference material 5.2a

Results

The study GPs enrolled 2078 patients; 1972 of these were sent appointments. No patient was lost to follow-up. Of those sent appointments, 106 patients (5.4%) failed to attend. Demographic details of the patients and information about their GP are shown in Table 1. The mean (standard deviation) referral rate during the study was 13.7 (6.3) per hundred patients per year. There were no significant differences in non-attendance between specialties. Men aged 16 to 35 years had a non-attendance rate of 21 %.

The univariable and multivariable results are shown in Table 2. Males, younger patients, those with a longer interval between referral and appointment, those with a higher Jarman score, and patients of a high-referring GP were all less likely to attend.

Table 1 Characteristics of non-attenders, compared with attenders and cancellations

Characteristic	Attenders and cancellations (n=1866)	Non-attenders (n=106)	Statistical test applied and significance
Percentage male (95% Cl)	40.2 (38.0–42.5)	50.9 (41.0–60.8)	χ^2=4.9 P=0.03
Mean age in years (95% Cl)	49.2 (48.1–50.2)	38.2 (34.2–42.1)	t-test=4.85 $P<0.0001$
Median (interquartile range) interval between referral and appointment (days)	50.7 (26.3–89.1)	110 (56.6–157.0)	Rank sum test $P<0.0001$
Percentage from a fundholding general practitioner (95% Cl)	23.9 (22.0–25.9)	29.2 (20.8–38.9)	χ^2=1.6 P=0.21
Percentage from a general practitioner with MRCGP[a] (95% Cl)	73.9 (71.7–75.8)	79.3 (70.3–86.5)	χ^2=1.5 P=0.22

[a] Membership of the Royal College of General Practitioners

Table 2 Multivariable analysis of characteristics of non-attendance

Characteristic	Univariable analysis		Multivariable analaysis	
	Odds ratio (Cl)	Significance	Odds ratio (Cl)	Significance
Male sex	1.60 (1.08–2.38)	0.02	1.65 (1.09–2.50)	0.02
Age	0.98[a] (0.97–0.99)	<0.001	0.98[a] (0.97–0.99)	<0.001
Jarman score	1.02 (1.01–1.03)	0.003	1.02 (1.01–1.03)	0.008
Interval to appointment	1.06[b] (1.05–1.08)	<0.001	1.07[b] (1.05–1.09)	<0.001
Referral rate of GP	1.03[c] (1.00–1.05)	0.06	1.03[c] (1.00–1.06)	0.05

[a] For a one-year increase in age. [b] For a one-week increase in interval. [c] For an increase of one referral per hundred patients per year.

Question 9   With reference to current evidence, discuss the effectiveness of the following interventions in management of stroke:

Stroke units
Surgery
Radiology
Drug treatment

Question 10 **While looking at ways to improve the care of patients with epilepsy in your practice, you come across the paper 'A pragmatic randomized controlled trial of a prompt and reminder card in the care of people with epilepsy' (*British Journal of General Practice* 2002; 52: 93–98; reference material 5.3a).**

Comment on the strengths and weaknesses of the method described.

Comment on the results of the trial (shown in Tables 1, 2 and 3 of reference material 5.3b)

Comment on possible reasons for these results

Reference material 5.3a

Method

Protocol

Practices in four areas of Greater Manchester (Stockport, South Manchester, Salford and Trafford, and Bury and Rochdale) were randomly selected and approached to participate in this study. The study was conducted between April 1997 and August 1999. Adults with 'active' epilepsy (either a seizure recorded in the medical records in the past two years or being on anticonvulsant medication for epilepsy) on the list of consenting GPs were eligible to participate. Temporary residents, individuals with severe learning disability, and children (individuals under 16 years of age) were excluded.

Intervention

The intervention consisted of an evidence-based epilepsy prompt and reminder card for GPs to complete. The card had two main parts: first, 'prompts' to collect key clinical information about an individual's epilepsy; and secondly, evidence-based information ('reminders') on which to then base any subsequent patient management decision. The final version of the prompt and reminder card was passport-sized, bright yellow in colour, and consisted of nine sections (including seizure frequency and pattern, seizure classification, medication, side-effects and indications for medication withdrawal, checking serum levels, information provision, and monitoring).

Assignment

The study was a pragmatic randomised trial. Practices were stratified into small (fewer than three partners in practice) or large (three or more partners in the practice). Using a random number table, practices were either allocated to the 'control' group, to the 'doctor-held card' group (where the card was inserted into the patients' records) or to the 'patient-held card' group (where the patient held the card). The card was used opportunistically over the course of one year for most subjects.

The primary outcome measures were recording of seizure frequency and self-reported seizure frequency in the previous year. Secondary outcome measures were the retrieval rate and completion rate of the epilepsy card, the proportion of patients on monotherapy with anticonvulsants, the proportion of patients reporting medication side-effects, whether serum levels of anticonvulsants were checked appropriately, the levels of patient satisfaction with GP care, and level of satisfaction with information provision by the GP.

The outcome measures used were items from the Liverpool Assessment Battery and information recorded in GP medical records. The Liverpool Assessment Battery comprises several scales (including the Seizure Severity scale, the HAD questionnaire) and individual items to measure the quality of life and the quality of care for people with epilepsy. Baseline questionnaire data were collected before randomisation with further questionnaire data being collected after the intervention. Data from medical records were extracted on two separate occasions (for baseline year and intervention year information).

Ethical approval was obtained from the relevant ethical committees (South Manchester, Bury and Rochdale, Salford and Trafford, and Stockport) prior to commencing recruitment.

Statistical methods

The sample size calculations were based on an estimated 10% reduction in seizure frequency and recorded seizure frequency (with 80% power and a 5% significance level). As randomisation was by practice, an intra-class correlation coefficient of 0.02 was estimated for outcome measures to account for clustering within practices. Previous studies had found that each GP had about 10 patients with epilepsy and that the average practice size was 3.5 GPs. It was calculated that 20 practices in the three arms of the study with 600 patients in each arm would yield enough power to detect this difference in seizure frequency.

Statistical analyses were based on generalised estimating equations, in which the intra-cluster correlation is accounted for using an exchangeable correlation model assuming a logistic model for binary outcomes. Prior to analysis, covariates that were potential predictors of outcome were identified and included in the model to improve efficiency and reduce chance bias. Analyses were carried out using the STATA statistical software. Where baseline covariates were missing, an additional 'missing' category level was used or an imputed value was assigned for continuous variables.

For each outcome, comparison was made between the three groups by means of a 0.05 two-tailed significance level using a Wald χ^2 test. Where there was evidence of difference between groups, pair-wise tests were carried out between the control and each of the intervention groups using a 0.025 two-tailed significance level. Analysis was done on an intention-to-treat basis.

Reference material 5.3b

Table 1 Recording of seizure frequency, either in medical records or on card in previous year

	Control	Doctor held	Patient held	Overall
Baseline				
In medical notes % (*n*)	37.8 (143/378)	36.6 (186/508)	36.5 (133/364)	37 (462/1250)
Intervention year				
Medical notes or card % (*n*)	42.8 (157/367)	57.4 (281/489)	44.6 (158/356)	49.3 (596/1210)
Adjusted[a] odds ratio relative to control group (95% CI)	–	1.82 (1.23–2.69)	1.16 (0.76–1.77)	
Wald χ^2 comparing intervention with control[a] (one degree of freedom)	–	$P = 0.003$	$P = 0.49$	$P = 0.0058$[b]

Intra-class correlation coefficient = 0.051.
[a] Adjusted for baseline recording of seizure, health problems, and visit to specialist in baseline year.
[b] Wald χ^2 comparing three arms (two degrees of freedom).

Table 2 Reported seizure frequency during the baseline and intervention year

Seizure status in previous year	Control	Doctor held	Patient held	Overall
Baseline year				
Seizure free % (*n*)	48.3 (181/374)	51.6 (247/479)	52,0 (179/344)	50.7 (607/1197)
intervention year				
Seizure free % (*n*)	51.5 (151/293)	56.0 (219/391)	58.1 (158/272)	55.2 (528/956)
Adjusted[a] odds ratio relative to control group (95% CI)	–	1.33 (0.83–2.13)	1.47 (0.88–2.46)	
Wald χ^2 comparing intervention with control[a] (one degree of freedom)	–	$P = 0.238$	$P = 0.137$	$P = 0.297$[b]

Intra-class correlation coefficient = 0.022.
[a] Adjusted for baseline seizure frequency, health problems, age, and visit to specialist in baseline year.
[b] Wald χ^2 comparing three arms (two degrees of freedom).

Table 3 Summary of other results on medication use, side-effects, and monitoring and on satisfaction with GP care during the baseline and intervention year

	Control	Doctor held	Patient held
Medication use			
On more than one epilepsy drug in baseline year % (n)	28.8 (106/368)	28.1 (131/467)	32.1 (110/343)
On more than one epilepsy drug in intervention year % (n)	28.9 (83/287)	30.3 (113/373)	29.9 (79/264)
Adjusted[a] odds ratio relative to control group (95% CI)	—	0.76 (0.41–1.44)	1.51 (0.74–3.07)
Wald χ^2 comparing intervention with control[a] (one degree of freedom)	—	P=0.401	P=0.253
Medication side effects			
Medication side effects reported by patient during baseline year % (n)	52.8 (182/345)	50.8 (229/450)	53.2 (173/326)
Medication side effects reported by patient during intervention year % (n)	43.6 (120/275)	49.3 (182/369)	50.8 (125/246)
Adjusted[b] odds ratio relative to control group (95% CI)	—	1.54 (1.10–2.17)	1.60 (1.10–2.32)
Wald χ^2 comparing intervention with control[b] (one degree of freedom)	—	P=0.013	P=0.016
Checking of phenytoin serum levels in previous year (for those patients on phenytoin)			
Phenytoin serum levels checked in baseline year % (n)	31.2 (39/125)	28.1 (52/185)	32.6 (42/129)
Phenytoin serum levels checked in intervention year % (n)	31.5 (34/108)	28.7 (45/157)	39.2 (40/102)
Adjusted[c] odds ratio relative to control group (95% CI)	—	0.93 (0.44–1.97)	1.37 (0.61–3.09)
Wald χ^2 comparing intervention with control[c] (one degree of freedom)	—	P=0.851	P=0.447
Satisfaction with information provision by the GP in previous year (for those patients who reported seeing the GP in the previous year)			
Satisfied with information provided by the GP in baseline year % (n)	67.7 (195/288)	64.4 (239/371)	65.1 (183/281)
Satisfied with information provided by the GP in intervention year % (n)	76.1 (175/230)	66.0 (195/295)	76.2 (162/213)
Adjusted[d] odds ratio relative to control group (95% CI)	—	0.57 (0.38–0.86)	0.98 (0.62–1.54)
Wald χ^2 comparing intervention with control[d] (one degree of freedom)	—	P=0.006	P=0.943
Rated GP care of their epilepsy as high (either excellent or good) (for those patients who reported seeing the GP in the previous year)			
Rated GP care of their epilepsy as high in baseline year % (n)	77.2 (223/289)	76.7 (284/370)	77.5 (217/280)
Rated GP care of their epilepsy as high in intervention year % (n)	79.0 (181/229)	73.6 (220/299)	83.6 (179/214)
Adjusted[e] odds ratio relative to control group (95% CI)	—	0.70 (0.45–1.07)	1.35 (0.80–2.21)
Wald χ^2 comparing intervention with control[e] (one degree of freedom)	—	P=0.10	P=0.27

[a] Adjusted for baseline number of epilepsy drugs. tonic clonic seizures. GP attendance's intervention year. [b] Adjusted for baseline presence of medication side-effects. other long-term illness. age. [c] Adjusted for baseline checking of phenytoin levels and age. [d] Adjusted for baseline information provision and age. [e] Adjusted for baseline satisfaction with care and age.

Question 11 Discuss the impact of deprivation on general practice.

Question 12 A 21-year-old girl and her boyfriend come for the morning-after pill. They both have Down's syndrome and attend a local daycare centre. What issues does this raise, and how would you proceed?

Paper 6

Question 1   Hannah, a normally fit and active 3-year-old, is brought to you by her parents. She is lethargic, dehydrated and smells ketotic. A fingerprick BM shows a blood glucose of 22. What are your aims now and in the future?

Question 2   'Growing old gracefully' – how can general practice meet the needs of elderly people?

Question 3   The NSF for Elderly People and Stroke places new emphasis on the prevention and treatment of stroke. See reference material 6.1a, an extract from the paper 'Use of ramipril in preventing stroke: double blind randomized trial' (with copyright permission from *British Medical Journal* 2002; 324: 699).

Comment on the methodology of the trial

Comment on the results in Table 1 of reference material 6.1b

Comment on the statement from the conclusion 'Widespread use of an angiotensin converting enzyme inhibitor such as ramipril in patients at high risk of stroke is likely to have a major impact on public health'

Reference material 6.1a

Design and methods

The HOPE study was a double blind randomised trial with a two by two factorial design, in which participants were randomised to receive up to 10 mg of ramipril, 400 IU of vitamin E, both, or matching placebos. We provide a brief outline here.

Participants

Participants were aged 55 or over and were at high risk of cardiovascular events because of previous coronary artery disease, cerebrovascular disease, or peripheral arterial disease or diabetes plus one additional risk factor. Patients were excluded if they were taking either an angiotensin converting enzyme inhibitor or vitamin E; had heart failure or a known left ventricular ejection fraction of less than 0.40, known proteinuria, or uncontrolled hypertension; or had had a previous stroke or a myocardial infarction less than one month before enrolment in the study. Informed consent was obtained from all participants before enrolment in the study, and the study was approved by the ethics committee at each centre.

Intervention

Eligible patients entered a run-in phase in which they received 2.5 mg ramipril daily for 7–10 days, after which serum creatinine and potassium levels were measured. Participants then started a 10–14 day course of placebo. Those who tolerated and adhered to this regimen were then randomised to receive either placebo or 2.5 mg ramipril daily for one week, followed by placebo or 5.0 mg ramipril for a further three weeks. One month after randomisation the patient's serum creatinine and potassium were measured; if these were satisfactory the patient continued on either placebo or 10 mg ramipril for the remainder of the study. Participants were seen after six months and then every six months until the end of the study, with an average follow up of 4.5 years.

Of the 10 576 patients who entered the run-in phase, 1035 were not randomised because of non-adherence, side effects, or withdrawal of consent; 244 patients were entered into a substudy of 2.5 mg ramipril and are not included in this paper. Outcome results were available on 9539 (99.9%) of the 9541 patients randomised. The first participant was recruited in December 1993. The originally scheduled completion date was November 1999, but the ramipril arm of the study was terminated early (April 1999) because of clear benefit.

Outcome measures

The primary outcome was the composite end point of myocardial infarction, stroke, or cardiovascular death. The individual components of this composite end point were analysed separately. All outcomes were adjudicated by a central committee. This analysis focuses on stroke.

Investigators reported the occurrences of stroke or transient ischaemic attack at follow up visits. For every stroke reported, information on the stroke, including symptoms and functional impairment, was documented. The investigators used a simple six point scale to record if there was full recovery, persistent symptoms, some functional impairment, functional impairment necessitating the assistance of others to perform activities of daily living, or inability to perform activities of daily living even with help at seven days or at discharge if earlier. Discharge summaries, consultation notes, and results of computed tomography or magnetic resonance imaging were documented. A central committee adjudicated all strokes on the basis of predetermined definitions. Classification of a stroke as either ischaemic or haemorrhagic was confirmed by computed tomography or magnetic resonance imaging within 14 days of onset or by autopsy. All other strokes were classified as being of uncertain aetiology. Computed tomography, magnetic resonance imaging, or autopsy results were obtained for 84% of strokes.

Blood pressure was measured at entry to the study, after two years, and at the end of the study. Two measurements were taken on each arm after the patient had been supine for five minutes. The lowest measurements on each arm were averaged to obtain the systolic and diastolic values that were recorded.

Statistical analysis

The study had 90% power to detect a 13.5% reduction in relative risk for the primary outcome, with an annual event rate of 4% in 9000 patients studied for five years. Assuming a stroke rate of 1.2% per year in the control group for five years, the study had 80% power to detect a 22.0% reduction in the relative risk of stroke with a two sided α level of 0.05 in an intention to treat analysis. We estimated survival curves according to the Kaplan-Meier procedure and compared treatments by using the log rank test. Because of the factorial design, we stratified all analyses for the randomisation to vitamin E or placebo. We conducted subgroup analyses by using tests for interactions in the Cox regression model. We used this model to estimate the reduction in relative risk and the 95% confidence intervals associated with ramipril treatment in unadjusted analyses and after controlling for changes in blood pressure.

The data and safety monitoring board monitored the study. Monitoring boundaries for the study were four standard deviations between the two groups in terms of benefit of ramipril in the first half of the study and three standard deviations in the second half. For harm, the boundaries were three standard deviations in the first half of the study and two standard deviations in the second half. Because of clear benefit, the study was terminated on 22 March 1999.

Study organisation

The study was conducted in 267 hospital clinics in 19 countries. It was coordinated by the Canadian Cardiovascular Collaboration in Hamilton, Canada.

Reference material 6.1b

Table 1 Impact of ramipril on stroke subdivided by non-fatal and fatal stroke, subtype of stroke, and presence or absence of functional impairment. Values are numbers (percentages) unless stated otherwise

Outcome	Ramipril (n=4645)	Placebo (n=4652)	Relative risk (95% CI)
Total strokes	156 (3.4)	226 (4.9)	0.68 (0.56 to 0.84)
Non-fatal:	139 (3.0)	182 (3.9)	0.76 (0.61 to 0.94)
No functional impairment	49 (1.1)	80 (1.7)	0.61 (0.43 to 0.87)
Some functional impairment*	85 (1.8)	108 (2.3)	0.78 (0.59 to 1.04)
Fatal	17 (0.4)	44 (1.0)	0.39 (0.22 to 0.67)
Subtype of stroke			
Ischaemic	101 (2.2)	157 (3.4)	0.64 (0.50 to 0.82)
Non-ischaemic†:	63 (1.4)	78 (1.7)	0.80 (0.57 to 1.12)
Haemorrhagic	12 (0.26)	16 (0.34)	0.74 (0.35 to 1.57)
Uncertain aetiology	52 (1.1)	65 (1.4)	0.79 (0.55 to 1.14)

* Any impairment from functional impairment that does not limit daily activities to assistance needed for all activities of daily living.
† Stroke of haemorrhagic or uncertain aetiology.

Question 4   The practice receptionist points out that there seem to be a large number of patients not attending appointments. What do you need to consider when looking at this problem?

Question 5   A 30-year-old woman with a BMI of 32 comes to see you requesting a prescription for slimming drugs which she read about in a magazine. What issues does this consultation raise?

Question 6   **With reference to recent literature, discuss the use of the following in primary care:**

Nurse practitioners
Community pharmacists

Question 7   Discuss the evidence relating to the following in the diagnosis and management of dementia:

Assessment
Drug treatments
Social care

Question 8   Discuss how doctors can identify their learning needs.

Question 9   One of your practice nurses wishes to go on a course on screening for prostate cancer. What issues does this raise and how would you address her request?

Question 10 **With regard to child health in primary care, comment on the following areas of controversy, giving evidence to support your views:**

Attention deficit hyperactivity disorder
- Diagnosis
- Treatment

Neonatal screening
- Deafness
- Congenital dislocation of the hip
- Cataracts

Question 11 (a) What are the problems encountered in studying therapies in arthritis?

(b) See reference material 6.2a, an extract from the paper 'Long term effects of glucosamine sulphate on osteoarthritis progression: a randomized, placebo-controlled clinical trial'. Reprinted with permission from Elsevier Science (*Lancet* 2001; 357: 251–256).

Comment on the methodology

Comment on the results in Tables 2 and 3 of reference material 6.2b

Reference material 6.2a

Methods

Study design and selection of patients

We recruited patients from the outpatient clinic of the Bone and Cartilage Metabolism Research Unit of the University Hospital Centre in Liege, Belgium. Inclusion criteria were age over 50 years and primary knee osteoarthritis of the medial femorotibial compartment, diagnosed according to the clinical and radiological criteria of the American College of Rheumatology. Disease severity was graded on the basis of the Kellgren and Lawrence radiographic system. Major exclusion criteria were: history or active presence of other rheumatic diseases that could be responsible for secondary osteoarthritis; severe articular inflammation as confirmed by physical examination (excluded also by erythrocyte sedimentation rate <40 mm/h and serum rheumatoid factor titre $<1{:}40$); traumatic knee lesions; overweight defined as a body mass index >30; substantial abnormalities in haematological, hepatic, renal, or metabolic functions; and intra-articular or systemic corticosteroids in the 3 months preceding enrolment. The study was approved by the ethics commitee of the University of Liege and all patients gave their oral and written informed consent to participate.

Treatment assignment

Crystalline glucosamine sulphate (Dona, Viartril-S, or Xicil, Rotta Research Group, Monza, Italy) is a defined pure substance that is synthesised from chitin, and in which glucosamine sulphate, chloride, and sodium ions are present in stoichiometric ratios of $2{:}1{:}2{:}2$. The net content of glucosamine sulphate in the dose form (powder for oral solution, with standard inactive excipients) is 1500 mg. This product has been approved at this once daily dosage as a prescription treatment for osteoarthritis in many countries in Europe and elsewhere.

Patients were randomly assigned to receive 1500 mg of glucosamine sulphate or placebo once daily for 3 years. For rescue analgesia, patients were allowed access to paracetamol in 500 mg tablets, or to one of the following NSAIDs (the most used in Belgium at the time of the trial): diclofenac in 50 mg tablets, piroxicam in

20 mg capsules, or proglumetacin in 150 mg tablets. Use of the rescue medications was recorded by the patients in a diary, with appropriate washout – ie, at least five half-lives of the selected medication were allowed before symptom assessment. Compliance with study treatment was established by asking the patients about missed doses and by counting unused sachets. No other co-interventions for osteoarthritis were allowed.

The randomisation list was generated by computer in blocks of four, and patients received their randomisation number in chronological order. The principal investigator was provided with individual envelopes, each containing patient codes, thus concealing treatment assignment.

Outcome measures

The primary outcome measure for joint structural changes was represented by the mean joint-space width of the medial compartment of the tibiofemoral joint. Weightbearing, anteroposterior, separate radiographs of each knee were taken at baseline, 1, and 3 years by a standardised technique. In brief, patients stood with their knees fully extended and the posterior aspect of the knee in contact with the vertical cassette. The lower limbs were rotated until the patella was centralised over the lower end of the femur. Feet were positioned a small distance apart: foot maps were used for repositioning the patient. The X-ray beam was centred on the joint space and parallel to the tibial plateau. Fluoroscopy was used to correct lower limb positioning and X-ray beam alignment. The focus to film distance was 110 cm.

We digitised the radiographs and did the image analysis automatically by a validated system, which located the proximal and distal joint margins excluding outlier points and calculated the mean joint-space width of the medial and lateral compartments of the tibiofemoral joint. We calculated the mean (SD) short-term and long-term coefficient of variation of this system for reproducing measurements as 1·82% (1·29) and 1·62% (1·31), respectively, for the medial compartment, which is in good agreement with the 1·84% coefficient of variation reported in the original validation of this method. All radiographs obtained in a single radiological unit in Liege were measured in London by a single reader unaware of treatment assignment. A further masked analysis was visual determination of the minimum joint-space width – ie, at the narrowest point – with a 0·1 mm graduated magnifying lens.

We assessed symptoms of osteoarthritis by the Western Ontario and McMaster Universities (WOMAC) osteoarthritis index, a validated, disease-specific questionnaire addressing severity of joint pain (five questions), stiffness (two questions), and limitation of physical function (17 questions), and referring to the 48 h before assessment. The visual analogue scale version of the index was used – ie, with the patient assessing each question by a 100 mm visual analogue scale, and the total index score being represented by the sum of the 24 component item scores. A higher WOMAC score represents worse symptom severity, with 2400 mm being the worst possible total score.

Secondary outcome measures were use of rescue medications as recorded in a daily diary; withdrawal rates; occurrence of adverse events; and routine safety

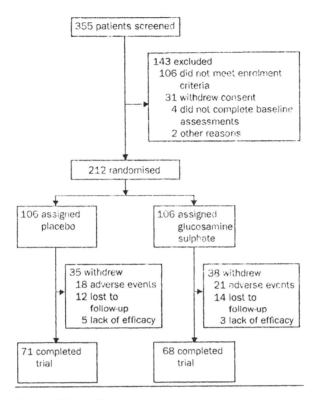

Figure 1: **Trial profile**

laboratory tests, including testing for glucose homoeostasis assessed by fasting glucose concentrations at yearly intervals in all patients still receiving the study treatment.

Statistical analysis

We calculated sample size on the basis of the recommendations available at the time of study planning, of a 0·5 mm target difference in joint-space narrowing between groups after 3 years, given the validation data of the digital image analysis technique adopted as the principal outcome. We calculated that a sample size of at least 60 patients in each group would give a power of 80% in detecting such a difference at the 5% significance level. We increased the sample size to at least 100 patients per group to allow an up to 40% dropout rate.

The primary efficacy outcome measure for structure modification was joint-space narrowing in the signal joint – ie, the change in joint-space width after 3 years in the narrowest medial tibiofemoral joint compartment at enrolment. The medial tibiofemoral joint space is preferred in clinical trials, as opposed to the lateral space, since this is the area that is subjected to the greatest pressure and thus the most osteoarthritis cartilage loss, and for which outcome measures are better validated. The 3-year % change in the total WOMAC score was taken for the primary assessment of symptom modification, with the final changes in the pain, physical function, and stiffness subscales analysed as secondary endpoints.

Results were expressed as difference between the final group means and 95% CI, with p values based on analysis of variance. All primary efficacy analyses were done on patients who completed the 3-year observation period, and by intention-to-treat analysis for all randomised patients. Every effort was made to carry out the final examinations after 3 years, regardless of patient's compliance or whether the patient was still on the study treatment. When this was not possible, the intention-to-treat analysis was carried out according to three different approaches. First, we did a worst scenario analysis in which a poor outcome was assigned to patients in whom the final 3-year assessment was not completed, corresponding to the average change recorded in patients in the placebo group who were assessed for 3 years. For consistency we also used the last observation carried forward approach, and to avoid repeatedly assigning the same value to a series of missing values we used the random sampling method. In the random sampling approach, missing endpoint values were replaced with values selected randomly from the distribution of all known endpoint values – ie, glucosamine sulphate and placebo combined. To lower sampling error, 50 such datasets were constructed, analysed independently by analysis of variance and the median of the significance values was taken.

Among secondary analyses, we arbitrarily defined a cutoff point for marked structural damage progression as a joint-space narrowing of more than 0·5 mm, based on previous reports – the proportion of all randomised patients reaching such a progression cutoff was compared between groups by the χ^2 test. The mean number of days of rescue medication intake was assessed by analysis of variance. We used the Spearman correlation test to assess correlation between structure and symptom outcomes. Adverse event and dropout rates were analysed by χ^2 or Fisher's exact tests, as appropriate. Baseline characteristics were compared by the χ^2 test for categorical variables and by analysis of variance for continuous data. All reported p values are two sided with $\alpha=0.05$.

Reference material 6.2b

Table 2 Average (95% CI) joint-space narrowing after 3 years

	Patients assessed for 3 years				Intention-to-treat analysis			
	Placebo (n=71)	Glucosamine sulphate (n=68)	Difference (95% CI)	p	Placebo (n=106)	Glucosamine sulphate (n=106)	Difference (95% CI)	p
Mean joint-space narrowing (mm)	−0.31 (−0.57 to −0.04)	0.07 (−0.17 to 0.32)	0.38 (0.02 to 0.73)	0.038	−0.31 (−0.48 to −0.13)	−0.06 (−0.22 to 0.09)	0.24 (0.01 to 0.48)	0.043
Minimum joint-space narrowing (mm)	−0.40 (−0.64 to −0.17)	0.11 (−0.10 to 0.33)	0.51 (0.20 to 0.83)	0.002	−0.40 (−0.56 to −0.24)	−0.07 (−0.22 to 0.07)	0.33 (0.12 to 0.54)	0.003

Table 3 Average (95% CI) total WOMAC percent change after 3 years

	Patients assessed for 3 years				Intention-to-treat analysis			
	Placebo (n=71)	Glucosamine sulphate (n=68)	Difference (95% CI)	p	Placebo (n=106)	Glucosamine sulphate (n=106)	Difference (95% CI)	p
Total WOMAC % change	9.8% (−14.6 to 34.3%)	−24.3% (−37.0 to −11.6%)	34.1% (6.4 to 61.8%)	0.016	9.8% (−6.2 to 25.8%)	−11.7% (−20.3 to −3.2%)	21.6% (3.5 to 39.6%)	0.020

Question 12 See reference material 6.3a, an extract from the paper 'The effect of
GP telephone triage on numbers seeking same day appointments'
(reprinted with copyright permission from *British Journal of
General Practice* 2002; 52: 390–392).

In terms of relevance to managing demand in UK general practice,
discuss the methodology and results of this study

Reference material 6.3a

Method

The study took place from July 1999 to June 2000 and was carried out in a group
practice located in a market town, with a list size of 7200, and four GPs. Levels of
deprivation were close to the national average (Jarman score = -4.26). The practice
introduced a telephone consultation policy whereby all patients requesting same-
day appointments were told that a GP would telephone them later. GPs were asked
to log the outcome of these telephone consultations. A patient satisfaction survey
was sent to all patients who had received such a telephone call over a one-month
period during the intervention. Numbers attending out-of-hours were compared
with previous years.

Statistical analysis

Numbers attending the surgery for routine and 'extra' appointments over two years
(1997 and 1998) were entered onto an SPSS database. Regression analysis was
performed to determine if there was a pattern to the demand for 'extra' appointments and if this pattern had a temporal basis. These data were used to assess the
impact of a telephone triage intervention. To determine the impact of the telephone
triage intervention, linear regression was performed on the logged counts with a
harmonic term to allow for seasonality and a dummy variable which takes the
value zero for pre-intervention and one for post-intervention. The analysis was
performed using autoregression in SPSS to allow for serial correlation and linear
regression using the Durbin-Watson statistic, to test whether serial correlation had
been successfully removed.

Results

A plot of the 'extra' appointments for 1997 and 1998 suggested a seasonal pattern.
A regression of the number of extra appointments required against time was
reasonably well fitted (adjusted $R^2 = 0.40$). A reduction of 39.3% in the demand for
face-to-face appointments was observed during the intervention phase as shown in
Figure 1.

Patient satisfaction survey

A 74% response rate to the postal questionnaire was recorded (111 responses in total). The majority of patients were satisfied or very satisfied with the outcome of the telephone consultation (98%) and most (84%) said they would be happy to receive this service in similar circumstances in the future (95% CI = 76 to 90). Patient use of out-of-hours services showed a drop in the study period.

Use of telephone

The total number of calls in the second half of the study period from January 2000 to June 2000 was 3680, with an average duration of less than two minutes. Ninety-three per cent had a duration of less than five minutes. The telephone bills increased by £200 per quarter over the study period. The total number of telephone calls recorded during one month in the second half of the study period was 615. The outcomes as recorded by the GPs in their telephone consultation diaries over this month are shown in Table 1 (outcomes not mutually exclusive, i.e. some telephone consultations resulted in more than one outcome).

Discussion

Our study suggests that it is possible to use telephone consultations as an alternative to face-to-face consultations for patients seeking same-day appointments. More than one in five patients were offered a prescription without a clinical examination, All patients receiving a prescription who responded to the questionnaire expressed satisfaction with the outcome of their telephone consultation.

The role of nurse practitioners for patients seeking same-day appointments or in telephone triage has been endorsed recently. However, the management of patients seeking same-day appointments in our study was streamlined by GPs without diverting nursing staff away from other roles. It has been argued that the increasing promotion of nurse practitioners to deal with patients who need a same-day appointment might promote inequality rather than improve primary care. This paper suggests an alternative for those who might wish to retain access to GPs on a same-day basis. However, there is a financial cost to offering this service, as the practice would have to pay more in telephone charges.

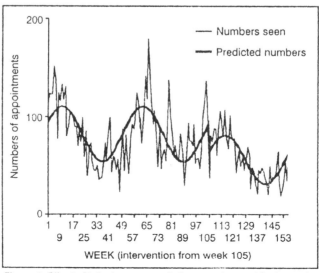

Figure 1. Effect of telephone consultations on demand for 'extras'.

Table 1 Outcome of telephone consultations

Outcome	Numbers (percentage of total)
Same-day appointment offered	266 (43.3)
Advice only	180 (29.3)
Prescription offered without face-to-face consultation	138 (22.4)
Visit	15 (2.4)
Routine appointment offered (not same day)	25 (4.1)
Appointment with nurse	8 (0.8)
Patient not available to speak to doctor	7 (1.1)

Part 3:
Answers

Paper 1

Answer 1   See reference material 1.1a, part of a paper entitled 'Meta-analysis of increased dose of inhaled steroid or addition of salmeterol in symptomatic asthma (MIASMA)' (Reprinted with copyright permission from *BMJ* 320; 1368–1373).

Comment on the outcome measures used

The outcome measures mentioned in the abstract are clinically relevant but imprecise. What is efficacy? Is it objective changes in peak flow or FEV, or subjective symptoms?

Comment on the methods for identifying suitable studies

- The researchers searched EMBASE, Medline and GlaxoWellcome databases, considering all studies in any language.
- Study search and selection was conducted by one person in isolation. Explicit criteria were used in the search. There is no mention in the methods of independent verification of screening, which may allow inclusion bias.
- All the studies included were sponsored by GlaxoWellcome. This may be coincidence, or may represent inclusion bias.
- Including the GlaxoWellcome database may remove publication bias if all clinical trials, i.e. including those that failed to show a significant effect, are represented. If, however, the database is selective it may introduce more bias. The GlaxoWellcome database is not externally reviewed, so we cannot know whether it is free from bias.
- The screening flow chart shows that the process of screening was relevant to the clinical question, i.e. comparing increased steroid to salmeterol.

Comment on the studies included

- The review suggests that it is looking at the question of increasing inhaled steroids from 100 to 400 µg of beclomethasone (50 to 200 µg of fluticasone) or adding salmeterol (step 3 of asthma guidelines, The British Guidelines on Asthma Management *Thorax* 1997; 52(Suppl 1); 51–52). The studies included, however, had a range of inhaled steroid doses from 200 to 1600 µg per day. Are these patients comparable, since they may represent very different groups of asthma patients, some of whom may not be at step 3 of the asthma protocol or equivalent?
- Separate analysis of groups by steroid type and dose may show whether there is a steroid-specific effect confounding the results.
- The studies are all large, which gives the systematic review sufficient power when they are pooled.

Comment on the results shown in Table 5 of reference material 1.1b

- The results of all the individual studies fail to show a benefit for salmeterol compared with increased steroids. Pooled results appear to show a small benefit for salmeterol, but the confidence intervals are wide and they approach the line of no effect. The p values given (0.79 and 0.85) are not statistically significant.
- The treatment effect is 2.73%, i.e. a number needed to treat (NNT) of 37.

Comment on the applicability of these results to clinical practice

These results fail to show any significant difference between the two therapeutic choices. Although this may not show that salmeterol is better, it does not show that it is worse. Steroids are not without side effects and it may be that salmeterol is a better choice at stage 3 of the asthma guidelines if it produces the same clinical effect with fewer side effects.

Answer 2

An 18-year-old model comes to you complaining of a 3-month history of amenorrhoea.

Outline your management

Amenorrhoea is a common problem, but in this consultation it is important to be empathic and ensure the patient feels listened to, with her concerns taken seriously.

History

Take full medical, menstrual and sexual history.

- Is she pregnant or using contraception?
- Any prescribed or illicit drug use, e.g. Depo-Provera, phenothiazines, amphetamines?
- What are her concerns/ understanding of the problem – worried about pregnancy/STDs/infertility/gynaecological disease?
- Why has she presented now – does a friend or family member have gynaecological or fertility problems? Any relationship difficulties?

Explore psychological issues, e.g. career pressures to maintain ideal weight or image causing eating disorders. Look for weight changes and purging or laxative abuse. The patient may resent questioning. Is she depressed? Is she happy in her job? Is she being sexually exploited?

Examination/Investigations

- Any evidence of excessive weight loss – BMI, lanugo hair, skin changes, electrolyte disturbance.
- Consider pregnancy and blood tests – usually after 6 months

amenorrhoea but if patient or doctor need reassurance, or there is suspicion from the history, check prolactin, LH/FSH, oestradiol, testosterone, TFTs.

Management

- Advise her about ideal weight, healthy eating habits, risks of excess weight loss.
- If she is pregnant, offer all options and support.
- This is an opportunity to discuss contraception. Tailor efficacy/side effects to lifestyle, e.g. avoid acne/weight gain with Depo-Provera. She may be happy not to have periods but you need to ensure she understands the need for contraception.
- Consider gynaecological referral if you suspect any abnormality. Consider osteoporosis prevention if there is prolonged oestrogen deficiency.
- If there is an eating disorder or psychological illness, consider referral to counsellor, CPN or specialist eating disorder service. Tailor treatment plan to lifestyle, e.g. psychotherapy may not fit in with travel and she may not engage.

Issues for the Doctor

- Potentially long, difficult consultation that may overrun. Consider review appointments.
- Potential awkwardness for male GP seeing attractive female patients; may feel more comfortable handing over to female colleague. How does the patient feel?
- Your own attitude to glamour industry may affect feelings – do you see it as exploitation? Do you have teenagers of your own with concerns about eating disorders?
- A patient who is pregnant and requesting abortion may cause ethical difficulties for the doctor.
- Any educational needs regarding amenorrhoea and eating disorders?

Wider Issues

- Eating disorders are increasingly prevalent. Be aware of signs to allow early identification and help.
- Need to educate PHCT. Consider literature or posters in practice, highlighting the problem and how to seek help.
- Need to lobby nationally against portrayal of thin as ' ideal' by the media and glamour industry.
- Improve provision of services for those with eating disorders – currently very patchy.

Answer 3   The father of an 8-year-old girl requests that you record and investigate his concerns that his estranged wife may have Munchausen's-by-proxy. What are the implications of this?

This situation encompasses a number of difficult issues and the response to the request needs to be carefully considered.

The implications can be categorised in the following way.

Implications for the Child

- Is she at risk?
- What would be the effect of bringing allegations out in the open? Will parental access be denied, exacerbating the emotional trauma of divorce? Will the child be subjected to unpleasant investigation to confirm or deny illness?
- What would be the emotional effect on the child of being used as a pawn?
- Genuine childhood illness may be untreated either because of the suspicion that her mother is fabricating symptoms, or because the mother fears being accused of fabricating illness.
- Who should consent to investigations on child to prove or disprove allegations?

Implications for the Father

- May be hostile if he feels he is ignored, may be worried about his children but feel unable to act.
- May be looking for evidence for custody battle.

Implications for the Mother

- Will need support and advice, whether or not allegations are true.
- Is the father trying to obtain confidential information about her?
- Genuine psychological problem may have been neglected.
- If the allegations are untrue, stigma may persist, resulting in considerable social problems, e.g. work.
- Investigating the allegations may cause a breakdown in relationship with the GP or health visitor.

Implications for the GP

- Very difficult case; you will need to be aware of your feelings and emotional state, e.g. fear of missed diagnosis.
- Is there an educational need? Review knowledge of Munchausen's.
- May be at risk of accusations of breach of confidentiality if reveals medical records of wife or daughter to father, or negligence if allegations are ignored but are true.
- Potential conflict of interest if you are also the mother's GP. Can you avoid taking sides?
- Consider need for medico-legal advice, e.g. from MDU.

Implications for the PHCT

- Health visitor may have a better relationship with mother than GP, although this may be a hindrance.
- Discuss with PHCT to ensure everyone is aware of allegations, and has a chance to air their thoughts.
- Do other members of the PHCT share concerns? If so, why have they failed to mention them before? Do they feel unable to air them?
- Good relations with social services to ensure appropriate organised and measured response.
- Is there an educational need for PHCT? Significant event meeting?
- Need to ensure everyone is aware of confidentiality issues.

Implications for Secondary Care

- May require paediatric or psychiatric input.

Answer 4   Mrs Bhatia is having hospital-initiated infertility treatment and attends for a repeat script. You note you wrongly prescribed her clomipramine last time instead of clomiphene. What issues does this raise?

Such incidents rarely happen in isolation. Investigating the accident chain allows us to install safeguards to prevent recurrence.

Consultation Issues

- Acknowledge guilt and embarrassment about the mistake.
- Avoid temptation to ignore incident and shrug responsibility.
- You need to be open and give a full apology to the patient and her partner (if present).
- The consultation may be long; consider a double appointment.
- Allow and encourage the patient to ask questions about what has happened. She may need to be offered more time at a later date.
- Be aware of language problems in explaining the mistake. Consider the use of an interpreter.
- Loss of trust in the doctor–patient relationship may follow. Full and frank apology may help.
- Is the patient pregnant? Review effects of clomipramine in pregnancy. If it is teratogenic you may need to consider referral for termination, and resulting emotional trauma.
- Housekeeping. Emotions may be drained, so take time before starting next consultation.

How has the Incident Happened?

- Has Mrs Bhatia taken clomipramine recently or in the past, remaining on the medication screen of the computer or repeat medications card if hand-held notes used?

- Has a typing or scanning error in outpatient notes been entered into the computer?
- If using a computer picking list, has the wrong drug been selected and prescribed in error by the doctor? Could it have happened with other patients?
- Has the patient presented with side effects of the treatment?
- Has she been referred back by the hospital who may be questioning compliance?
- Have language or communication problems played a part?
- Cultural factors may contribute, e.g. the patient notices the error but her cultural background prevents her questioning the doctor.
- Stress may cause lack of concentration by the doctor.

Medical Issues

- Need to consider potential effect of clomipramine on other medications e.g. FSH, side effects, and any withdrawal effects.
- Need to inform fertility specialist. This will be professionally embarrassing and will affect future interactions with them.
- Consider need to review prescribing of unusual drugs initiated by specialists, e.g. interactions and side effects.

Ethical Issues

- Non-malificence. Ensure she stops the clomipramine and check for harm as a result of treatment.
- Beneficence. Start correct medication and ensure appropriate follow-up. Is she aware of the side effects of fertility treatment?
- Confidentiality. She may or may not wish the mistake to be discussed with family members.
- Social justice. Should fertility treatment be available in a resource-limited NHS?

Patient Issues

- She may be worried about harmful effects now or in future pregnancies.
- Advise her on complaints procedure.
- Has she suffered other mistakes in the past, because of cultural or communication barriers?
- She may not trust the GP in the future.

Medico-legal Issues

- Review contemporaneous notes and contact MDU.
- Inform the other partners and practice manager of what has occurred.
- If patient unhappy, encourage formal complaint to show that her concerns are properly addressed.
- Take immediate steps to prevent recurrence.

Practice Issues

- Significant event audit should establish causation and prevent recurrence. Should be supportive, not punitive.
- Staff need to be sympathetic to Mrs Bhatia and her family. They may be keen to consult for explanations and be given an opportunity to do so. They may need to be given appointments at short notice.
- Prescribing should be reviewed, particularly if there has been an error in a repeat prescription or as a result of a computer 'pick list'.
- Consider review of complaints procedures; are they easy for all ethnic groups to understand?
- Need for adequate medico-legal record in case of legal action.
- Support the doctor. Error has occurred. Offer time off if stressed, or time for personal development.
- Consider mentoring.
- Discuss with dispensing pharmacist. Did he notice the change in prescription? Is there any potential safety net at this level?

Answer 5 Comment on the following treatments for the menopause, under the headings Factors and Comments and Evidence:

Factors	Comments and Evidence
HRT	
Use of HRT:	A population survey in Wandsworth found that South Asian women were significantly less likely to take HRT (1).
Breast cancer:	Small excess risk associated with HRT in meta-analysis, risk disappears within 5 years of stopping (2). Risk may be greater with combined treatment, with excess risk of 25–40% at 5 years (3, 4).
Heart disease:	In HERS 4, the Heart Estrogen/progestin Replacement Study (5), 52% increase in cardiovascular events in the first year of therapy in patients with a history of heart disease on HRT. At 4 years there was no overall difference. The oestrogen replacement and atherosclerosis trial (6) of women with coronary stenosis found no significant change in angiograms compared with placebo. The Women's Health Initiative (7) primary prevention trial, showed an excess of myocardial infarction in the treatment group. In 2001 the American Heart Association reversed earlier advice to use HRT in patients at risk of heart disease.
Colon cancer:	Meta-analysis suggests the risk of colon cancer is reduced by one-third in current and recent users of HRT (8).
Dementia:	Some epidemiological studies show delayed onset and progression of Alzheimer's disease (9), although there was possible selection bias towards educated people in the treatment arm.

Factors	Comments and Evidence
Bone:	A Swedish trial of HRT and hip fracture (10) showed protection during treatment and for a few years afterwards. Continued protection needs continued use. A meta-analysis of all fractures concluded that there was a protective effect but the NNT was 40.
Thromboembolism:	Research using the General Practice Database shows a 2-fold increase in idiopathic DVT, mostly in the first year of use (11).
SERMs	
Menopausal symptoms:	*Clinical Evidence* (12) concludes that tibolone is effective for menopausal symptoms. May be helpful if the patient cannot take oestrogen.
Lipids:	Evidence suggests raloxifene lowers cholesterol levels (13).
Bone:	*Drugs and Therapeutics Bulletin* (14) found raloxifene to be effective in preserving bone mass.
Phytoestrogens	A *Bandolier* review (15) found RCT evidence that phytoestrogens in soya beans caused a 40% reduction in vasomotor symptoms.

References

1. Ethnic differences in use of hormone replacement therapy: community based survey. *British Medical Journal* 1999; 319: 610–611
2. Breast cancer and hormone replacement therapy: collaborative reanalysis of data from 51 epidemiological studies of 52 705 women with breast cancer and 108 411 women without breast cancer. *Lancet* 1997; 350: 1047–1059
3. Menopausal estrogen and progestin replacement therapy and breast cancer risk. *JAMA* 2000; 283: 485
4. Hormone replacement therapy and the breast. *British Medical Journal* 2001; 323: 1381
5. Randomized trial of estrogen plus progestin for secondary prevention of coronary heart disease in postmenopausal women. Heart and Estrogen/progestin Replacement Study (HERS) Research Group. *JAMA* 1998; 280(7): 605–613
6. Effects of estrogen replacement on the progression of coronary artery atherosclerosis. *New England Journal of Medicine* 2000; 343: 522–529
7. National Institutes of Health, National Heart, Lung, and Blood Institute. Women's Health Initiative. Available at: www.nhlbi.nih.gov/whi/hrt-en.htn
8. Hormone replacement therapy and the risk of colorectal cancer: A meta-analysis. *Obstetrics and Gynecology* 1999; 93: 880–888
9. Cognitive function in nondemented older women who took estrogen after menopause. *Neurology* 1998; 50: 368–373
10. Hormone replacement therapy and risk of hip fracture: population

based case-control study. *British Medical Journal* 1998; 316:
1858–1863

11. Hormone replacement therapy and risk of venous thromboembolism:
population based case-control study *British Medical Journal* 1997; 314:
796

12. *Clinical Evidence*, Issue 7 (August 2002); Section: Women's Health,
Menopausal Symptoms.

13. Effects of raloxifene on serum lipids and coagulation factors in healthy
postmenopausal women. *JAMA* 1998; 279: 1445–1451

14. Raloxifene to prevent postmenopausal osteoporosis. *Drug and
Therapeutics Bulletin* 37(9); 24–25

15. Alternatives for the menopause. *Bandolier* 56; Volume 5, Issue 9, 3–4

Answer 6   Your practice is considering setting up a sleep clinic for parents of
children with sleep problems. Read reference material 1.2a, an
abstract from the paper entitled 'Randomised controlled trial of
behavioural infant sleep intervention to improve infant sleep and
maternal mood' (Reprinted with copyright permission from *British
Medical Journal* 324; 1062–1065).

Comment on the strengths and weaknesses of the methodology

Research Question

Addressed a clearly focused question, relevant to general practice.

Population

- Only looked at children aged 6–12 months, these problems are common
and perhaps more significant in older children. Are the results
generalisable? The control and intervention groups were broadly similar.
- Selection of participants through routine child health screening should
give a good representative sample of mothers. Exclusion of those with
poor English may make the study less applicable to the general
population.

Intervention

Intervention is described but impossible to say if it was standardised e.g. by
following a protocol.

Outcome Measures

- Outcome measures were a mixture of objective Edinburgh Postnatal
Depression score, which is a validated and accepted measure, and
maternal report of sleep problem (yes/no), which is subjective and open
to recall bias.
- Analysis was on an intention-to-treat basis, making the results
generalisable to the clinical setting.

Sources of Bias

- The study was not blinded. The participants were randomised to control or intervention and masked at the analysis stage, which should reduce bias in analysis.
- The intervention was significantly different from that received by the control group. It would have been better to have given the control group three sessions of 1 to 1 consultation as well, but not given specific advice about sleep. This would have removed the possibility that it is the process of having 3 sessions with a friendly supportive professional that is beneficial rather than the advice about sleep.
- Inclusion criteria were maternal report of sleep problem and objective evidence of sleep problems, while at follow-up presence of sleep problems was a subjective yes/no. Some mothers may consider it normal for children not to sleep through the night, hence answer no to the question.

Statistical Methodology

- Sample size calculated to ensure power. The numbers of patients in the trial exceeded this number.
- Used regression models, a validated method of analysis.

Comment on the results shown in reference material 1.2b

Participant Flow and Follow-up

Only 232 out of 738 who completed the survey were eligible to participate, and 155 agreed to do so. The description of the two groups lists 78 participants in each, i.e. 156 subjects. No mention of subjects who do not appear in follow-up, i.e. total of 152 participants at 2 months and 146 at 4 months. Were these missing people admitted to psychiatric hospital or did they commit suicide? Impossible to tell.

Significance of Results

- The results show that more control mothers reported sleep problems and needed extra help at 2 months, with p values of 0.005 and 0.006, both of which are statistically significant.
- At 4 months, the differences were not significant (p = 0.26).
- The results for depressive scores only became significant after they were adjusted to account for additional professional help. This may bias the result. The results as reported were significant, with narrow confidence intervals.

Answer 7   How could you improve the care of teenagers?

Teenage healthcare is challenging: they visit surgeries infrequently, and may mistrust services. Drug misuse, psychological morbidity including depression, suicide and eating disorders are important problems, and reducing teenage pregnancy is one of the government's Health of the Nation targets.

Factors to consider in planning teenage healthcare services include the following:

Identifying Needs

- Involve teenagers in planning, e.g. questionnaires on needs and how to make practice appealing, or approach local school/youth groups to ask teenagers directly.
- Hold competition to design practice posters to give sense of ownership.
- Liaise with local school nurses to ascertain what services they feel are required.
- Use available evidence on strategies tried nationally to improve uptake of services.
- Audit certain areas, e.g. pregnancy or termination rates, parasuicide rates, to identify areas of need.

Accessibility

- Appointments to suit their needs e.g. out of school hours or lunchtimes.
- Choices of personnel, e.g. instead of registered GP offer another GP or nurse.
- Consider offering them same day access to increase attendance.
- Be more flexible if late for appointments – inform receptionists.
- Inform patients about alternative ways to seek advice e.g. telephone, e-mail, NHS Direct.
- Consider open or walk in sessions for young people, perhaps run informally (e.g. by casually dressed staff) in evenings or Saturday mornings.
- Consider outreach health education sessions by doctors or nurses at schools or youth groups.

Promoting the Practice and Resources Available

- Need to make teenagers feel that they are welcome and their needs are appreciated.
- Consider colourful, prominent posters in waiting room or on practice door stressing confidentiality and outlining services available, e.g. contraception, sexually transmitted diseases.
- Easily accessible leaflets on e.g. eating disorders, sexual health plus prominently displayed contact numbers for services such as Family Planning clinic, GUM clinic, and teenage advice phonelines.
- Ensure all staff are welcoming to teenagers who attend – do not ask too many questions when they book appointments, etc., and respect their privacy.
- Liaise with school nurses to ensure awareness of services available.

- Supply free condoms.

Practice Staff Issues

- All staff need to be up to date on specific health needs of teenagers particularly contraception, advice on unwanted pregnancy, drug abuse. Receptionists should be aware of when to offer rapid access, e.g. for emergency contraception. May need training sessions. Utilise paediatric, psychiatric or family planning staff as resource and update regularly.
- Ensure list of local resources available for teenagers accessible to all staff.
- Help all practice staff to feel comfortable dealing with young people. Teenagers may be seen as aggressive, abusive or disrespectful but this may be a sign of fear or uncertainty. Ensure staff feel supported and safe. Consider training sessions on how to approach this age group.
- Stress importance of confidentiality.

Resource Issues

- A lot can be achieved with minimal financial outlay but may entail costs in staff time; some plans (e.g. dedicated clinics) are expensive.
- Teenage health is a government health priority, so funds may be available. Successful pilots could be expanded to other practices.
- Diverting energies to teenage health may reduce resources available elsewhere, e.g. for the over 75s.

Assessing Success

- Audit attendance rates and health outcomes (e.g. pregnancy).
- Consider patient satisfaction questionnaires to see if changes have been well received and identify areas for improvement.
- Staff meetings to discuss any problems and praise successes.

Answer 8   Mr Green and his wife come to see you for the result of his endoscopy. This showed an inoperable gastric carcinoma. How would you proceed, and what issues would you aim to cover?

Consultation Considerations

Before the Consultation

- Be fully informed, particularly regarding treatment options. Review latest hospital reports.
- Allow plenty of time, and avoid disturbances.

During the Consultation

- Avoid euphemisms and abbreviations. Be clear and concise, short and simple
- Find out what they know, what they fear and what they want to know.
- Encourage their thoughts and questions on the diagnosis and treatment.

- Allow plenty of time and let them dictate the pace of the consultation and have tissues ready.
- Find out how much they want their friends and families to know.

After the Consultation

- Arrange to see them again when the news will have sunk in, and be available for telephone advice.
- Advise practice staff and out-of-hours providers of situation should they be called about the patient.
- Consider support services such as CancerBACUP.
- Be aware of your own emotions after the consultation.

Issues to Cover with Mr and Mrs Green

Medical Issues

- Be prepared for them to ask about second opinions and the possibility of alternative treatments.
- Medical needs at present? Pain? Anaemic or cachectic? Depressed?
- Be vigilant for medical and psychological complications.
- Explore their ideas, concerns and expectations regarding cancer.
- If chemotherapy is an option, explore ideas, e.g. about hair loss.
- When appropriate, ask Mr Green what he wants to know about the end, and how he envisages it. Is he terrified of pain, or breathing problems?
- What are his aims? One last family holiday? Encourage realism, but support these aims.

Aims of Treatment

- Explain aims of treatment: physical and psychological support, avoid suffering and preserve dignity.
- Encourage positive attitude towards palliative care, explain role of hospice and arrange for palliative care nurse to contact them if they wish.

Social Issues

- Ensure social security support, e.g. attendance allowance. Any financial concerns?
- Assess housing needs, e.g. stair lift or rehousing?
- Need help with nursing?
- Encourage Mr Green to make a will, and consider an advance directive.

Psychological Issues

- Prepare Mr and Mrs Green for inevitable grief reaction. Support them through this.
- Encourage openness with family members, especially estranged ones. This may prevent pathological grief later.

Other Issues

- Keep an open mind about complementary therapies, e.g. reflexology.
- Need for hospital/hospice at-home service in the area?

Answer 9   Outline your strategies for dealing with difficult patients.

In attempting to understand difficult patients attempts have been made to categorise them, e.g. the dependent clinger, the entitled demander. Difficult patients are better thought of as one half of a difficult consultation and we must look to ourselves for some of the answer.

Understanding the causes of 'difficult' patients helps us to deal with them.

Doctor Factors

- We may promote patient anxiety or dependence by arousing unreasonable expectations, by unnecessary follow-up or through extensive investigations of minor problems.
- Our inability to identify physical symptoms of somatisation of a psychiatric illness may lead is to label these patients as 'difficult'.
- There is some evidence suggesting that overworked GPs and those who lack higher professional training and particularly training in consultation skills report more 'difficult 'patients.
- Where doctors feel ill-equipped to manage a condition, e.g. through lack of knowledge, they may find consultations with these patients difficult.
- Patients labelled 'difficult' by colleagues may bias our approach to the consultation.
- Our failure to understand family or social dynamics may cause mutual frustration.
- Finding patients 'difficult' may represent burnout in the doctor.

Patient Factors

- Complex problems often combined with difficult social circumstances may mean that patients are frustrated when we are unable to solve all their problems.
- Difficult requests or unrealistic expectations of the doctor or the health system.
- Unconventional health beliefs and non-compliance with treatment.
- Language or cultural barriers.
- Inappropriate health-seeking behaviour e.g. frequent attendance or unnecessary visits, a history of complaints or litigation may cause us to label them difficult.
- Patients who 'shop around' different doctors or surgeries with their symptoms are frequently seen as difficult.

Ethical Issues

- Justice: we should not let prejudice influence us, but equally we are the guardians of healthcare resources. Excessive referral, investigation or

treatment of demanding patients may deprive others.
- Beneficence: these patients may have genuine unidentified pathology that we should seek.
- Non-malificence: we must protect our difficult patients from harm, e.g. from unnecessary treatments.
- Autonomy: we should respect patient's views about their treatment, even if different from our own.

Strategies for Coping with Difficult Patients

For the Doctor

Tailor to the different characteristics of the patient but essentially:

- Recognise your own feelings towards the patient. 'Housekeeping' before or after the consultation before you can continue with the next patient.
- Take each consultation at face value to avoid missed diagnoses.
- Recognise temptation to investigate or refer as a result of doctor anxiety or pressure.
- Sharing the problem with colleagues within the practice, mentors or in Balint groups.
- You may need to be honest and open with the patient and share feelings of frustration with them.
- Go through old notes and review diagnoses for unrecognised illness.
- Consider a contract for patients who are abusing the system or medication.
- Videotape analysis of consultations may be beneficial and highlight problem areas in communication.
- Try modifying health-seeking behaviour. Time spent in explanation or education may be beneficial in long term.
- Develop strategies for patients with lists, e.g. limit of two problems per consultation.
- Be aware of stress or burnout and address this.

Practice Issues

- Aggressive patients require a staff policy. Staff safety is vital. Do rooms have panic alarms?
- Staff should be informed of difficult patients and discuss them.
- Practice policy for contracts or removal from list as a last resort.
- If relations have broken down, it may be in the patient's best interests to consult another doctor in the practice or consider a move to a different surgery.
- Consider significant event audit where appropriate.
- Involve the wider family or social network where appropriate.

Answer 10   With regard to end of life decisions, what are the arguments for and against ending life, withdrawing treatment and 'do not resuscitate' orders?

Right to Die

There are three situations:
- a person who wishes to kill themself but is physically unable to do so.
- a person who makes an advance directive regarding future treatment.
- a mentally competent person who wishes life-sustaining treatment to be withdrawn.

The GMC are currently drawing up explicit guidelines for doctors in these situations.

General Ethical Considerations

- Beneficence: aim to ease suffering.
- Non-malificence: does maintaining life prolong suffering? Is withdrawing treatment/assisted suicide causing pain?
- Autonomy: is the right to self-determination paramount in matters of life and death? Who decides for those unable to decide for themselves? Also includes previously expressed wishes regarding death.
- Social justice: should resources be diverted from life-saving treatments to life-prolonging treatments?

Assisted Suicide

- Assisted suicide is illegal in the UK. Diane Pretty, who had motor neurone disease, argued unsuccessfully that this blanket ban violated her right to life and other rights under the European Convention on Human Rights, arguing that the right to life included the right to end one's life.
- A similar High Court case was settled out of court when all sides agreed that under the doctrine of double effect, doctors may administer drugs to relieve physical and mental pain in the final stages of a severe degenerative disease, even if this shortens life.
- A *British Medical Journal* editorial 2001 (1) argued that the moral distinction between a mentally competent woman refusing life-sustaining treatment and requesting assistance with suicide is arbitrary.
- In Holland assisted suicide was decriminalised in 2001. Doctors must report to regional committees of doctors, lawyers, and ethicists, who check they have acted with due care, and if so close the case.

Withdrawal of Treatment in Mentally Competent Person

In 2002 the High Court allowed a quadriplegic patient to have her ventilator disconnected, ruling that competent patients had 'an absolute right to refuse to consent to medical treatment for any reason, rational or irrational, or for no reason at all, even when that decision may lead to his or her death'.

Advance Directives

These are legally binding, allowing patients to give or withhold specific consent prospectively. Surveys showed only 49% of GPs (2) were aware of this, and only a quarter of hospital trusts had policies for them. Should be made when mentally competent, witnessed, and state explicitly that their consequences should not preclude basic care. To deliberately ignore them is a criminal offence.

Withdrawal of Life-sustaining Treatment from Patients in a Persistent Vegetative State

- The patient cannot contribute to discussions on their care, as discussed in the *British Medical Journal* (3).
- There have been 20 cases so far in the UK. The legal justification is that patients must consent to any treatment they receive; patients in a persistent vegetative state (PVS) cannot legally consent and can be treated only if it is in their best interests. The question of whether life-prolonging treatment or care is in their best interests can be referred to the courts. In every case they have decided that it is not, and given permission to stop treatment.
- BMA guidelines (4) state that life cannot be preserved at all costs, treatment must be a benefit not burden, that nutrition and hydration are a medical treatment, that competent patients may refuse treatment, that where patients cannot express their opinions previously expressed wishes should be taken into account, and that there should be independent clinical review.
- Arguments against withdrawal are that the diagnosis of PVS is subjective, that there is no standard test of awareness and data on prognosis are limited. Increasingly the courts are considering patients whose lack of awareness is less clear-cut. Where is the line drawn?
- The High Court has ruled that article 2 of the Human Rights Act, which places a positive obligation on the state to safeguard life, does not apply to withdrawal of treatment in PVS.

'Do Not Resuscitate' Orders

Research by Age Concern suggests these are rarely discussed with patients and are used inappropriately by some staff because of ageism (5). Explicit guidelines from the BMA, Resuscitation Council and RCN state that they should always be discussed with the patient or others close to them. They should not result in substandard care in other areas. Evidence from the US suggests they are used more often in black people, alcoholics, non-English speakers, and people infected with HIV, suggesting prejudices over who is worth saving.

References

1. Why active euthanasia and physician assisted suicide should be

legalised. *British Medical Journal* 2001; 323: 1079–1080
2. Do general practitioners know when living wills are legal? *Journal of the Royal College of Physicians of London* 1998; 32: 351–353
3. Ethical issues in diagnosis and management of patients in the permanent vegetative state. *British Medical Journal* 2001; 322: 352–354
4. *Withholding and withdrawing life-prolonging treatment.* BMA 1999
5. Do not resuscitate decisions: flogging dead horses or a dignified death? *British Medical Journal* 2000; 320: 1155–1156

Answer 11   Discuss the evidence regarding the effectiveness of the following interventions in the primary care management of diabetes:

Glitazones

- Glitazones work like metformin by sensitising tissues to insulin. In addition they increase the HDL levels in the blood. Side effects include weight gain (1).
- When used with insulin, substantial falls in insulin requirement are reported, although cardiac failure may occur in this situation.
- Licensed as add-on second line therapy with metformin or sulphonylureas.
- They are cytochrome P450 inducers, so may interact with the pill. Contraindicated in liver impairment.

Universal Screening

- The NSF for diabetes states that 'The NHS will develop, implement and monitor strategies to identify people who do not know that they have diabetes.'
- The arguments for screening are that it is common, is an important public health problem, that many patients have complications at diagnosis, that a reliable treatment exists and will effect disease prognosis if instituted early (UK PDS (2), DCCT (3)), i.e. it fulfils many of the Wilson and Junger criteria.
- One proposed strategy is to screen everyone over the age of 45 with a triennial fasting blood glucose (American Diabetes Association).
- Arguments against this are that it would be expensive in time and resources, and will screen the worried-well rather than high-risk groups. An alternative is to target those at risk, e.g. the obese, hypertensives, and people with a strong family history. A trial of universal screening in primary care detected positive results in 0.2% of those with no risk factors, but 2.8% in high-risk groups (4).

Antihypertensives

- The UK Prospective Diabetes Study (2) comparing aggressive treatment of hypertension with atenolol or captopril with controls found a reduced risk of fatal and non-fatal macrovascular complications, and a 32% reduced risk of death, while microvascular complications were reduced by 34–47%.

- Subgroup analysis of the SHEP-91 study showed a 54% reduction in MIs (5).
- The British Hypertension Society Guidelines (based on the HOT study (6)) suggest an optimal blood pressure of less than 130/80 in diabetics.

References

1. Thiazolidinediones for type 2 diabetes. *British Medical Journal* 2000; 321: 252–253
2. Tight blood pressure control and risk of macrovascular and microvascular complications in type 2 diabetes: UK PDS 38. *British Medical Journal* 1998; 317: 703–713
3. The effect of intensive treatment of diabetes on the development and progression of long-term complications in insulin-dependent diabetes mellitus. *New England Journal of Medicine* 1993; 329: 977–986
4. Screening for diabetes in general practice: cross sectional population study. *British Medical Journal* 2001; 323: 548
5. Prevention of stroke by antihypertensive drug treatment in older persons with isolated systolic hypertension: final results of the systolic hypertension in the elderly program (SHEP). *JAMA* 1991; 265: 3255–3264
6. Effects of intensive blood pressure lowering and low-dose aspirin in patients with hypertension: principal results of the Hypertension Optimal Treatment (HOT) randomised trial. *Lancet* 1998; 351: 1755–1762

Answer 12   Read reference material 1.3a, taken from a paper entitled 'A controlled trial of sustained-release bupropion, a nicotine patch, or both for smoking cessation' (Reprinted with copyright permission from *New England Journal of Medicine* 340; 9: 685–692).

Comment on the strengths and weaknesses of the methodology

- The study addressed a clearly defined question and compared the three treatment options of patches, bupropion or both against placebo.
- Subjects were recruited by media advertisements. Non-English-speaking people were excluded, potentially reducing the generalisability of the results. Subjects were screened according to a set protocol, reducing inclusion bias. Allocation was randomised but method is unclear. Only smokers of more than 15 cigarettes a day were included, so results may not be applicable to lighter smokers.
- The intervention was standardised. The study was double blinded, with all groups having either placebo or real patches and tablets. Regular biochemical monitoring of indices of smoking may have reinforced the intervention, making it less applicable to a primary care setting, but this was also true for the placebo group.
- All participants were included in analysis of outcome, i.e. on intention-to-treat, making the study more relevant to clinical care. The follow-up

was of sufficient duration to detect real behavioural change.
- Outcomes were assessed as a point prevalence of not smoking at 6 or 12 months, confirmed by objective measurement of carbon monoxide in expired air. This is taken to confirm continuous abstinence by the researchers, but could mean only recent abstinence. It is not clear if the participants were aware in advance of the date of follow-up.
- Statistical analysis is by an accepted and validated method. The sample size was calculated prior to the study.

Comment on the data in Tables 1 and 2 of reference material 1.3b

- Baseline characteristics are essentially similar, except for the significantly higher number of other smokers in the household for the placebo group. They also had higher average daily consumption and expired carbon monoxide. These may make them less likely to give up.
- Subjects who were lost to follow-up or left the treatment were classified as smokers, consistent with an intention-to-treat methodology.
- Nicotine patches were not shown to be significantly effective, with odds ratios of 1.2 (0.7–1.9, $p = 0.53$) at 6 months and 1.1 (0.6–1.8, $p = 0.84$) at 12 months.
- Bupropion alone and in combination with patches was effective with odds ratios of 2.3 (1.4–3.7, $p \leqslant 0.001$) and 2.7 (1.7–4.4, $p < 0.001$) at 6 months respectively, and 2.3 (1.4–3.9, $p < 0.001$) and 3.0 (1.8–4.9, $p < 0.001$) at 12 months.
- The results suggest that nicotine patches are ineffective, although the wide confidence intervals and low p value suggest this result may be different in a larger trial population.
- The significance of the efficacy of combination therapy is unclear. If bupropion is effective on its own, then addition of anything to it would show combination therapy to be effective.

Paper 2

Answer 1 A 45-year-old businessman consults you because he has problems getting an erection. Discuss your management.

- Erectile dysfunction is a common problem, affecting as many as 39% of 40-year-old men, although only a small number of them consult their GP. There are many causes, both organic and non-organic.
- In this consultation the GP should recognise the difficulties a man may feel when presenting with such a sensitive problem. You need to be empathic, acknowledge his concerns and reassure him about confidentiality.

History

- Take a full history. What does he mean by erectile problems? Is this new? Does he have problems initiating or sustaining erections? Early morning erections? Does he masturbate?
- Review his medical history. Does he have diabetes, vascular or neurological disease? Is he a smoker or have a heavy alcohol intake? Is he taking prescribed or illicit drugs, e.g. antihypertensives?
- Look for hidden agendas, e.g. concern about heart or neurological disease.
- Does he have signs of psychological illness, e.g. depression or anxiety.
- Explore psychosocial context, e.g. relationship problems.
- Are cultural or religious beliefs affecting his sex life?
- Why has he presented now? Is he in a new relationship? Is he worried about fertility or STDs causing his problems?
- Explore his health belief model/ideas, concerns and expectations. What does he want out of consultation? Reassurance, drugs or referral?

Examination/Investigations

- For female GPs, consider chaperone/referral to male colleague for examination.
- Check BP, BMI and genitalia, looking for signs of disease including vascular disease. Check urine for glucose.

Management

- If signs of medical disorder treat accordingly, avoiding medication which will worsen problems where possible. Adjust medication if this is contributing. Advise on lifestyle modification, e.g. smoking.

- If psychological problems – offer to see with partner. Consider referral for psychosexual counselling. Avoid presumptions about sexuality.
- Discuss treatment options. Is he suitable for sildenafil – if he doesn't meet criteria for FP10 prescribing (e.g. diabetes, neurological disorders, pelvic surgery) would he pay for private prescriptions?
- Alternative treatments possible, e.g. Caverject. Consider referral to urologist.
- Ensure he feels supported and confirm understanding.
- Offer information about support groups.

Other Issues

For the Doctor

- Sensitive and potentially embarrassing topic – how comfortable do you feel in consultation? Do you yourself suffer with sexual problems and have struggled to seek help?
- If female, would you prefer to refer him to a male colleague – patient may prefer female.
- Maybe unfamiliar about impotence management options – may highlight learning need.
- You may have opinions about using drugs such as sildenafil. Is it a 'lifestyle drug' or an example of government rationing?

For the Practice

- Are surgery hours convenient for working patients?
- Are patients asked about reasons for consultation when booking appointments? This could deter those with sensitive problems. Advertise in reception/practice leaflet that reason does not have to be given.
- Ensure all staff are aware of confidentiality issues.
- Promotion of men's health e.g. specialised men's clinics. Use all opportunities for health promotion when men attend, both in consultations and with leaflets e.g. about testicular self-examination, etc. Directly question men in diabetic or cardiac clinics about impotence.

For Society

- Impotence is a major, largely hidden problem causing psychological morbidity. It should be considered as important as other illnesses. Needs adequate funding.
- Why do only certain illnesses allow for NHS prescriptions while others are rationed?
- Limited availability of trained psychosexual counsellors.

Answer 2 'You can't teach an old dog new tricks.' How can GPs stay up-to-date, and what are the risks and benefits of this?

GPs have a professional and a moral obligation to ensure they are fit to practice, and this includes a need to keep up to date. There are many ways of doing this, each with their costs and benefits.

Why do we Need to Keep Up-to-date?

- Duty of care to patients – need to be able to show that we are practising good medicine.
- Professional self-regulation relies on doctors being able to show that we are up-to-date.
- A GP who knows that he is up-to-date will have more self confidence.
- GPs receive incentive payments for demonstrating that they are keeping up-to-date.

How can GPs Keep Up-to-date and What are the Risks and Benefits of This?

Attendance at Educational Meetings

Advantages

- Aimed at GPs, with structured format, expert speakers and relevant material. Easy to quantify time spent on educational activity.
- Educational resources (e.g. handouts) provided, saving time in researching information.
- Cost may be offset by drug company sponsorship.
- Sociable. Attendance offers an opportunity to meet like-minded individuals, share problems and experiences and relax away from surgery.
- Can be lunchtime or evening meetings, avoiding impact on surgery.

Disadvantages

- Often lecture-based, hence often minimal audience participation.
- 'Experts' may not tailor content to general practice.
- Often expensive.
- Need for locums to cover duties disadvantages single-handed and rural GPs who find it difficult to get locums.
- Confirmation of attendance does not confirm understanding or benefit.
- May choose subjects they enjoy, rather than areas of educational need.
- Sponsorship may introduce bias.
- Disadvantages the geographically isolated, who cannot attend evening meetings.

Personal Learning Plans

Advantages

- Allow targeting of specific learning needs.
- Require active participation in learning.
- Encourage innovative learning e.g. the internet, as well as more traditional methods.

- Less attendance at meetings; more suitable for GPs who struggle to leave the surgery.
- Encourage reflective learning.
- Cheaper than attending a series of lecture courses.
- Having a mentor is supportive for stress of general practice as well as learning.
- Encourages a rolling process of reflection and review of goals.
- Easy to do, e.g. with PUNS and DENS to stimulate problem-based learning.

Disadvantages

- What to put in? No universal format. May be subjective.
- May be time consuming to prepare.
- May disadvantage those with less access to information technology.
- Based on a reflective learning style. Failure to acknowledge areas of need may just result in a plan to attend lectures in a favourite area, as above.
- Goals may be set low to ensure success.
- May increase professional and social isolation.

Clinical Attachments

GPs may choose to spend a session in outpatients to improve skills in that area.

Advantages

- Experience of secondary care management of conditions.

Disadvantages

- Difficulty tailoring to specific learning needs.
- Outpatient experience may be irrelevant to primary care.
- May be seen as an extra pair of hands rather than a supernumerary.
- Attendance does not mean improvement.

Reading Journals

Advantages

- Easy to do, anywhere, any time.
- Many journals are available on the internet.

Disadvantages

- Cost of journals.
- Impossible to read everything. Danger in being too selective.
- May read interesting articles, rather than those that may address a need.
- Time.

Answer 3   A 45-year-old secretary complains of intermittent loss of sensation in her left hand. You know her father has multiple sclerosis. How would you proceed?

Symptoms of sensory loss have a number of different causes including carpal tunnel syndrome, cervical spondylosis, and peripheral nerve lesions.

Patient Factors

- Is she aware of her father's condition?
- Likely to be anxious and worried.
- Needs to feel her concerns are taken seriously during the consultation and that she has been listened to.
- What are her ideas, concerns and expectations about her father's problems and potential diagnoses?
- Try to relate them to her psychosocial context with respect to her job, family, hobbies, etc. What type of secretary is she? What is the impact of her symptoms on her home/working life?
- This visit may be a plea for help for her father, or reflect hidden agenda, e.g. if sole carer not coping.

Consultation Issues

- Doctor may be apprehensive if not confident about neurological conditions and examination.
- Patient may be well informed, which may influence the outcome or choice of management.
- Review symptoms, e.g. distribution of paraesthesia, any other symptoms, e.g. neckache, diplopia, precipitating factors.
- Allow time to express her ideas and outline specific concerns by using open questions, reflection, etc.
- Consider psychological causes, e.g. anxiety and panic attacks causing paraesthesia.
- Open questions about family history give an opportunity to discuss her father.
- Do not assume concerns relate to her father's problems. She may not associate these symptoms and may be more concerned about carpal tunnel syndrome or repetitive strain injury.
- Share findings and likely diagnoses, putting them in context of concerns and agree a management plan.

Examination/Investigation

- Perform full examination relevant to differential diagnosis including CNS, CVS, fundi and neck.
- Tailor investigations to concerns. Consider ESR, glucose, TFTs, B_{12}, folate.
- If she has specific concerns about MS or suspicious findings consider a neurological opinion.

Management

- If symptoms suggestive of carpal tunnel consider simple treatment possibly with a splint or injection.

- If any other conditions identified, e.g. diabetes, treat accordingly.

Follow-up

- If no definitive diagnosis possible be honest, rather than bluffing.
- Arrange follow-up to allow review of progress and reporting of evolving symptoms.

Ethical Considerations

- Patient autonomy: Aim for informed, shared decision-making.
- Non-malificence: Investigations may increase concern and anxiety, or have side effects.
- Benificence: Appropriate treatment and or referral where indicated.
- Respect confidentiality regarding both her and her father's illness when dealing with either of them.

Other Issues

- Does the practice have a carers register – if caring for her father she should be on this.
- May qualify for disability living allowance if looking after her father.
- Multiple Sclerosis Society may help with father or daughter if she has the condition.
- Any educational needs for the doctor?

Answer 4   Discuss the use of referral rates in general practice with reference to the literature.

The unique role of GPs in the NHS as both patient advocate and gatekeeper has raised the possibility of reducing secondary care costs by concentrating on referral rates.

Referral rates are unsatisfactory indicators of quality because they hide failures to refer as well as unnecessary referrals. Patients may be harmed if referral occurs too late and delay can lead to more major treatment being required at a later stage.

How and Why do Referrals Vary?

Referral rates are reported to vary by 3–4-fold between GPs.

Doctor Factors

- GPs who dislike uncertainty or perceive serious disease to be more frequent refer more patients (1).
- Doctors with more experience in an area may be more aware of therapeutic options and refer more.

Patient Factors

A survey of referrals in Nottinghamshire (2) found deprivation accounted for 23% of the variation.

Other Factors

There is some evidence that when waiting lists come down, referrals to that service go up.

Are Referrals Avoidable?

- A study of 170 consecutive referrals from 1 GP suggested 1/3 were potentially avoidable if alternative resources had been available, e.g. lack of CPNs. Many avoidable referrals are due to insufficient knowledge or experience of the GP (3).
- Admission rates seem to correlate well with referral rates, implying that referrals are appropriate (4).
- A systematic review in 2000 (1) concluded GP and patient characteristics explained less than 50% of the variation, and that guidelines had limited effect.

How can Referral Rates be Modified?

Feedback
Feedback of referral rates is ineffective, largely because of scepticism that they are a marker of poor quality.

Guidelines

- In March 2002 NICE published referral guidelines for GPs. They have been criticised as being rather simplistic.
- A trial of referral guidelines for infertility concluded that these made a small difference to referral practices but no change in outcomes or costs (5).
- A review in *Family Practice* (1) concluded that rather than targeting high or low referrers through clinical guidelines, activity should concentrate on increasing the number of appropriate referrals, regardless of the referral rate. Pressure on GPs to review their referral behaviour through the use of guidelines may reduce their willingness to tolerate uncertainty and manage problems in primary care, resulting in an increase in referrals to secondary care.

Education

- Educational packages for doctors in management of menorrhagia reduced referral rates for hysterectomy, and increased the number of patients treated appropriately with hormonal therapy (6).
- Trials of education of patients suggest that when given evidence-based information regarding surgery for prostatism they are less likely to want referral (7).

Money
Increasing the provision of minor surgery in primary care under fundholding uncovered new demand, with minimal effect on secondary care (8).

References

1. Variation in GP referral rates: what can we learn from the literature?. *Family Practice* 2000; 17: 462–471
2. The effect of deprivation on variations in general practitioners' referral rates: a cross sectional study of computerised data on new medical and surgical outpatient referrals in Nottinghamshire. *British Medical Journal* 1997; 314: 1458
3. Avoidable referrals? Analysis of 170 consecutive referrals to secondary care. *British Medical Journal* 1994; 309: 576–578
4. Relation between general practices' outpatient referral rates and rates of elective admission to hospital. *British Medical Journal* 1990; 301: 273–276
5. Pragmatic randomised controlled trial to evaluate guidelines for the management of infertility across the primary care–secondary care interface. *British Medical Journal* 2001; 322: 1282
6. Randomised controlled trial of educational package on management of menorrhagia in primary care: the Anglia menorrhagia education study. *British Medical Journal* 1999; 318: 1246–1250
7. The effect of a shared decision-making program on rates of surgery for benign prostatic hyperplasia. *Medical Care* 1995; 33: 765–770
8. Prospective study of trends in referral patterns in fundholding and non-fundholding practices in the Oxford region, 1990–4. *British Medical Journal* 1995; 311: 1205–1208

Answer 5   The senior partner in your practice has the largest prescribing bill in the health authority. What are the implications of this and how would you approach the situation?

GPs are under increasing pressure to curb prescribing costs. There are a number of difficult issues that need to be considered in this situation.

Implications for the Senior Partner

Prescribing Issues

- Is he/she frequently away (e.g. on Primary Care Trust work), so locums are prescribing in his name?
- Is he/she prescribing inappropriately? Is this an indication of a wider problem?
- Is he/she generally a high prescriber or are certain drugs (e.g.proton pump inhibitors) prescribed frequently?
- Is the prescribing bill high because of brand prescribing rather than generic?
- Are his/her patients different from those of other GPs, e.g. special interest in HIV with patients on expensive drugs?
- Is he/she an enlightened prescriber with superior knowledge of therapeutics, using drugs rather than referral for other treatment modalities, e.g. PPIs rather than referral for surgery in reflux?

- Is he/she following the NSFs to the letter?

Interpersonal issues

- How is he/she likely to respond to discussion of prescribing habits?
- Is there a forum where discussion of prescribing may take place in a safe environment, e.g. monthly prescribing meeting?
- Does he/she acknowledge that there is a problem?
- Why has this become an issue now? Has he/she upset someone at practice or health authority?

Implications for Partners

- May be financial penalties if practice exceeds its drug budget, affecting development funds and profits.
- Clinical governance issues: if there is genuine concern about the senior partner the practice must act, to prevent future charges of negligence.
- Has situation arisen through a lack of clinical governance, e.g. no regular prescribing reviews?
- Discussion of these issues may provoke distrust and hostility, with implications far beyond prescribing.
- Is there a problem with repeat prescribing in general, e.g. failure to review medications regularly?

Implications for Primary Healthcare Team and Practice Staff

- Pharmacist: Involving a pharmacist in prescribing meetings and analysing PACT data may suggest areas for rationalisation and savings, e.g. changing to generics or using cheaper drugs from similar classes (e.g. lansoprazole rather than omeprazole).
- Practice manager: Needs to keep on top of the situation, including liaising with health authority.
- Receptionists: They are the interface between doctors and patients in any change in prescribing. They need to know how and why any changes are being made.

Wider Implications

- Health authority drug overspends may require savings elsewhere, e.g. closure of community hospitals.
- Patients: Are patients being denied the best treatment for a condition to save money?
- Doctors: Increasing use of guidelines impinges on professional autonomy. Conflict of interest between patient advocate and gatekeeper of NHS resources, increased by prescribing incentives.

Management of this Situation

- Arrange a meeting with partners to discuss prescribing when all can attend.
- Ensure all stakeholders feel they have ownership of process and agree aims of prescribing review.

- Look at everyone's prescribing – what can you learn from each other?
- Agree how prescribing review will be conducted, e.g. one section of the BNF at a time.
- Agree who will participate, e.g. pharmacist, one partner responsible for each section of BNF.
- Agree timetable for review and ensure aims auditable.
- Consider developing a practice formulary from review.

Answer 6   A 41-year-old ex-serviceman asks for help. He complains of palpitations, nightmares and work difficulties. He smells of alcohol. His wife has seen you about relationship difficulties. Outline your approach to this problem.

This situation represents a number of challenges and potential obstacles.

Consultation Style

- Requires open, unhurried style. Be aware that he may feel uncomfortable discussing personal issues.
- Respect confidentiality of all parties, especially consultations with wife about their relationship.
- Be aware of possible mental illness but also possibility of negative attitudes and stigma. Need to approach this carefully.
- Need to be aware of problems experienced by ex-servicemen.

History

- What are his principal complaints? What does he mean when he says he needs help?
- What are his ideas about his symptoms? Does he fear he has a serious heart condition?
- What are his concerns? Does he fear mental illness or Gulf War Syndrome?
- What are his expectations? Referral, reassurance or a sick note?
- Review symptoms, onset and treatments taken? Is he self-medicating with alcohol or other drugs?
- Is there a clear onset, e.g. after discharge, or traumatic incident? Ask about symptoms of PTSD.
- Any previous history of physical or mental health problems?
- Put complaints in a social context. Is he unemployed? On benefit? Has his wife threatened to leave him if he doesn't seek help?

Examination

- Aim to confirm or dispel any potential diagnoses, e.g. heart and blood pressure to reassure about these.
- Examine for general health. Any signs of alcoholism?
- Perform mini-mental state examination, looking for signs of depression.

Investigations

- Consider ECG, 24 hour tape and blood tests to rule out organic causes.

- If concern about alcohol consumption, consider checking LFTs.

Summarise and Hand Over

- Explain findings to patient and differential diagnosis.
- Offer written information on diagnoses and seek his opinions, especially if differential includes mental health problems.
- Offer early review by telephone or appointment to discuss concerns.
- Encourage him to bring his wife or a friend with him next time if he wishes.
- Agree a mutually acceptable approach to his problems. If appropriate suggest relationship counselling.

Management

- If PTSD likely, refer to psychiatrist.
- If depressed, consider drug treatment or referral for counselling.
- If excessive alcohol consumption, try and agree a realistic approach to reducing this.
- Suggest Royal British Legion for advice and support.
- If taking benzodiazepines, agree conditions for future prescriptions. Explain need to avoid dependence. Consider use of contract.

Other Issues

- Any learning needs, e.g. PTSD?
- Need to be available for review and support.
- Danger of doctor dependence, if patient sees GP in a paternal role previously supplied by the armed forces.

Answer 7   Your practice is considering providing a complementary medicine service to your patients. You wish to make the decision evidence-based. What are the difficulties in researching complementary therapies such as acupuncture? Comment under the headings below:

Study design

- The gold standard is the double blind randomised controlled trial. For many complementary therapies this is not feasible.
- In acupuncture, for example, sham treatments generate problems since they may not be a true placebo. Patients cannot be effectively blinded, since it is obvious that they are having acupuncture, not placebo.
- The practitioner often cannot be blinded because of the nature of complementary therapies.
- Many complementary therapies are labour intensive, which may make it very difficult to obtain data on enough patients to provide adequate statistical power.
- Objective outcomes for studies in complementary medicine are difficult to quantify, leading to reliance on subjective ones such as wellbeing, which are prone to bias.

Bias and confounding

- The process of treatment may be a significant confounder, e.g. reflexology may be very pleasurable, resulting in enhanced wellbeing separate from any supposed effect on the body's inner workings. This causes problems both in choosing objective outcome measures and in eliminating confounders.
- These studies are prone to inclusion and exclusion bias, since patients often have fixed beliefs about the relative efficacies of treatments and will select therapies they believe in (self-inclusion bias). Complementary therapists may be less likely to offer treatments to people they believe are sceptics.
- There may be problems with standardising treatments. Many complementary therapies, e.g. homeopathy, are tailored to the individual and hence individual treatments cannot be compared in the way antibiotics might be. Another source of bias is that for many complementary therapies there may not be standardised training, so an acupuncturist in Croydon may be practicing totally differently from one in Liverpool.
- It may be difficult for practitioners to be objective and avoid unintentional bias, since they usually have strong faith in their own therapy.

Results

- There may be problems extrapolating results from individual trials to the general population. Both the therapist and the patients studied may be significantly different from the population seen in general practice.
- The data may not be amenable to standard statistical analysis, with heterogenous outcomes and low sample numbers. This makes it difficult to compare either between individual complementary therapies or between them and conventional medicine.
- These studies are less amenable to meta-analysis than conventional research for the same reasons: heterogeneity and lack of standardisation.
- Recent trials of homeopathic treatments for allergy failed to show any clinical effect. Homeopaths defended their treatments, arguing that as each individual is treated according to their unique make up and individual problem. Two individuals receiving homeopathy for the same problem cannot be compared, let alone two treatment arms in a large study.

Answer 8   See reference material 2.1a, taken from the paper 'A single blind trial of reflexology for irritable bowel syndrome' (Reprinted with copyright permission from *British Journal of General Practice* 2002; 52: 19–23).

Comment on the strengths and weaknesses of the methodology

- The study aimed to answer a clearly defined question, to examine the efficacy of reflexology in the management of the core defining symptoms of IBS.
- The study was single blinded. Double blinding would not be possible since the practitioner cannot administer the treatment blind.
- The study had tight inclusion criteria: all patients diagnosed with IBS in accordance with the Rome criteria, a validated classification. They had all been diagnosed by a gastroenterologist, which would remove alternative diagnoses, e.g. Crohn's disease, which may confound.
- Patients with new symptoms, i.e. those who may spontaneously improve, were excluded, as were those who had previously had reflexology, to avoid them knowing whether they were having reflexology or placebo. The use of patients with chronic symptoms only potentially removes any effect of increased attention alone.
- Patient selection was via a notes search, followed by randomisation by alternation, but the numbers in each group are different: this is not accounted for in the methods and may represent bias in randomisation.
- The numbers of patients involved are small and although sample size was calculated, this was not reached, reducing the statistical power of the study.
- Control and treatment groups received identical treatments but it is not clear from the method whether they all received treatment from the same person or whether there was a standardised treatment protocol for the actual treatment rather than just a standardised process.
- Outcomes were assessed with a standardised assessment tool, reducing subjective bias in outcome reporting. Statistical assessment was by a validated method.

Comment on the results shown in reference material 2.1b

- 100% of randomised patients were followed up at the end of the treatment and 83% at 3 months.
- Baseline characteristics are given and are essentially the same.
- The fact that participants who were questioned about their treatment and who guessed did so correctly may suggest that blinding was inadequate, but 2/2 may be coincidence because the sample size was so small.
- None of the outcomes measured shows a statistically significant result, although confidence intervals and p values are not given. The range of results is wide and an effect might become apparent with larger populations.

Answer 9   Your practice is considering becoming paperless. What considerations may surround this decision?

Computers are an invaluable tool in general practice, facilitating record keeping and information flow, and we are being encouraged practically and financially to become paperless.

Benefits to Practice

- Records legible and less storage space required.
- Increased data accessibility, less likely that information lost.
- Helps avoid errors – repeat prescribing, highlighting of allergies or drug interactions.
- Use for reminder systems, e.g. cervical smear recalls or annual blood tests.
- Templates for consultations, e.g. contraception or new patient checks.
- Possible direct link for IOS claims.
- Facilitates audit.
- Allows use of tools for consultation, e.g. decision support software for nurse-led clinics, or e-mail consultations.
- Access to internet for education or patient information leaflets.
- Software for e.g. anticoagulation allows delegation of work to other staff members.
- Will facilitate flow of information between providers, e.g. to secondary care or out-of-hours service.

Making the Decision

- Need to ensure all feel involved in planning; ownership aids acceptance.
- Ensure all staff understand benefits but listen to concerns, e.g. increased workload. Staff may be resistant to change, needing reassurance, adequate training, support and practical transition.
- Ensure regular meetings for problem solving.
- Have clear schedule for implementation. Will it be completely paperless, or will hospital letters/results remain as hand-held notes? Is scanning equipment required? Will a pathology link exist for results from local hospital?
- Needs clear plan – consider staggered introduction.
- Funding? Grants may be available to purchase system and training costs, but may divert resources from other services.
- Consider compatibility with PCT/hospital systems, e.g. pathology links.

Implementing System

- Will take time for staff to learn new skills. Cover must be arranged during this period.
- May leave practice short-staffed, resulting in increased stress, dissatisfaction or errors.
- Consider extra pay, time off in lieu or practice away-day.
- Consider training providers, e.g. computer company or health authority.
- Aim training at needs of different groups of staff with opportunities to practice, ask questions and feedback.
- Consider nominated IT co-ordinator to whom problems can be referred.
- Need computers to practise on, either in practice or at outside venues.
- Consider visiting other practices with systems in place.

Potential Problems

- Any system is only as good as the information put on it.
- Transferring data on to system is time-consuming – needs dedicated staff.
- Need to adhere to Data Protection Act. Enforce confidentiality issues.
- May slow down consultations initially. Patients may dislike computers.
- Sensitive information on screen visible to family members attending with patient. Confidentiality concerns.
- Temporary staff (e.g. temps or locum GPs) may be unfamiliar with system. Ensure clear information or training available, e.g. details in locum packs.
- Difficulties for branch surgeries or home visits. Will need print outs and manual entering of details on return. Laptop computers a possibility, but expensive.
- Risk of viruses, or hackers accessing confidential records – ensure adequate security system.
- If system fails, need rapid access to specialist help. Ensure practice has contingency plan.
- Will it be suitable to meet future national targets, e.g. electronic patient records, or need replacing in few years?

Answer 10   A 38-year-old with knee pain informs you during the consultation that her husband is clinical director of the local hospital. What considerations affect the consultation, and how would you proceed?

This situation requires careful consideration and delicate management.

Considerations for the Doctor

- Good rapport is essential. You may expect a difficult or long consultation.
- The patient may have specific ideas, concerns and expectations, and will almost certainly have had an informal opinion from her husband before seeing you.
- You may feel a 'messenger' in the referral process but may have to accept this.
- You may well be irritated by the mention of her husband if you feel she is using this to influence you.
- Important not to assume medical knowledge and take things at her pace.
- Why has she mentioned her husband's position? This suggests you may not be her usual GP; why is she not seeing them?

Ethical Considerations

- You may feel your autonomy about the management of the problem is threatened and may believe that the patient's husband will scrutinise your actions.
- You may need to reassure her regarding confidentiality.
- Can she get fair and impartial treatment at the hospital where her husband is the lead clinician?
- Social justice: referral should be based on need. There may have to be

more room for negotiation if she has fixed expectations, although her expectation may be a private referral.

- Non-malificence: inappropriate referral may result in unnecessary arthroscopy with possible risks.
- Benificence: if she has a genuine problem this must be addressed.

Consultation and Management

- Take full history for possible diagnostic cues.
- Any other joint problems?
- Explore psychosocial context – what are her job and hobbies? A forthcoming special event?
- Does her husband know she has come? This should not be assumed. Has he made a tentative diagnosis or suggested to her a particular course of action?
- Summarise what worries her most and her thoughts on the likely diagnosis before examination.
- Perform an appropriate examination of the knee and other joints if required.
- Consider offering a chaperone for the examination.
- Handover: Clear explanation in appropriate language about the likely diagnosis and management options, tailored to her ideas and concerns.
- Agree a mutually acceptable management plan. Is conservative management with analgesia appropriate? Are investigations required? Does this fit in with her expectations?
- Safety netting: Arrange follow-up.

Other Issues

- If referring, it is important to include her husband's position in the letter as this may assist the next person who sees her in their consultation.
- Access. If not consulting with her regular GP, why not? Are the appointments booked? Did she feel the usual GP would be unhelpful e.g. for a referral?
- Consider patient information leaflets on knee and other joint pain for simple physiotherapy or analgesia.
- Physiotherapy: does the practice have access to physiotherapy?
- Does the practice need to look at how doctors and their families are cared for by the practice, e.g. confidentiality regarding notes and practice staff access to these?
- Any learning needs?

Answer 11   What are the challenges in managing dyspepsia? Discuss the evidence under the headings below:

Investigations

The main challenge is to detect life-threatening conditions such as gastric cancer and peptic ulceration without subjecting patients with benign conditions to unnecessary investigation or treatment.

Two main clinical decisions are whether to endoscope or to test for *Helicobacter pylori*. The evidence/guidelines to guide in this decision are:

- NHS Guidelines for 2 week suspected cancer referrals:
  Urgent upper GI endoscopy if:
  – dysphagia
  – dyspepsia at any age with weight loss, anaemia or vomiting (1)
  – dyspepsia in patient >55 years old with recent onset or continuous symptoms
  – dyspepsia with risk factors, e.g. Barrett's oesophagus, family history
  – jaundice or upper abdominal mass.
- In absence of alarm symptoms, early endoscopy is unlikely to be helpful (2). Trial of lifestyle measures and antacid suggested for 4 weeks before considering endoscopy.
- Policy of testing for *H. pylori* followed by antibiotics in those who test positive is as effective as endoscopy, although fewer patients are satisfied with their treatment (3).
- In patients under 55, with uncomplicated dyspepsia, non-invasive testing for *H. pylori* is as effective, safe and reassuring as endoscopy, and less uncomfortable and distressing (4).

Treatment

Acid Suppression

- NICE guidelines: Clear benefits in some conditions. Start with cheapest at a healing dose, then step down as patients improve clinically. Use PPIs for NSAID-induced ulcers in people who must continue NSAIDs, those with severe GORD, those with ulcers who have not responded to a test and treat approach. All other patients should start with lifestyle advice/antacids/alginates, then H2 receptor antagonists, then PPIs.
- There is concern in some quarters about a rapid rise in prescriptions for PPIs. Estimated that if NICE guidelines were universally applied this would save £40–50 million per annum. A study of patients' and GPs' attitudes towards PPIs suggests that idea of profligate prescribers and lifestyle drugs is wrong; most patients are elderly, with complex health needs (2).
- There are concerns that use of PPIs before endoscopy may mask early gastric cancer. Suggested no patient over 45 should have a PPI before an endoscopy (5).

Eradication of *H. pylori*

- Gold standard is the breath test, with good sensitivity and specificity, normalising quickly after eradication.
- Eradication is indicated for non-NSAID-associated gastric and duodenal ulcers (6), non-ulcer dyspepsia and NSAID-associated ulcers where *H. pylori* infection is proven (7). It does not make reflux better.

- Treatment failures due to rapid development of resistance. Persistent symptoms may require re-testing or re-treating (6).
- A study suggests that eradication rates are higher in those who drink alcohol, compared with those on the same regime who do not (8).

Surgery

In severe GORD if PPIs fail to suppress symptoms, but there is some debate about the merits of laparoscopic rather than open fundoplication (9).

References

1. Dyspepsia in primary care – to prescribe or to investigate? *British Journal of General Practice* 2001; 51: 612–614.
2. Proton pump inhibitors: perspectives of patients and their GPs. *British Journal of General Practice* 2001; 51: 703–711
3. *Helicobacter pylori* test-and-eradicate versus prompt endoscopy for management of dyspeptic patients: a randomised trial. *Lancet* 2000; 356; 455–460
4. Randomised trial of endoscopy with testing for *Helicobacter pylori* compared with non-invasive *H. pylori* testing alone in the management of dyspepsia. *British Medical Journal* 2002; 324: 999
5. Proton pump inhibitors may mask early gastric cancer. *British Medical Journal* 1998; 317: 1606–1607
6. ABC of the upper gastrointestinal tract. *British Medical Journal* 2001; 323: 1047–1050
7. Role of *Helicobacter pylori* infection and non-steroidal anti-inflammatory drugs in peptic-ulcer disease: a meta-analysis. *Lancet* 2002; 359: 14–22
8. *European Journal of Gastroenterology and Hepatology* 2002; 14: 291–296
9. Laparoscopic or conventional Nissen fundoplication for gastro-oesophageal reflux disease: randomised clinical trial. *Lancet* 2000; 355: 170–174

Answer 12   Personal Medical Services (PMS) or General Medical Services (GMS)? Discuss the pros and cons of the contractual options for general practice.

Traditionally the GMS contract was the only option. Recently a proposal for an updated GMS contract has been unveiled together with a second option of PMS contracts.

Current GMS Contract

Key Points

- Nationally negotiated, i.e. applies to all GPs regardless of location
- Central funding through mixture of allowances, capitation and item of service fees.

- Earnings essentially unlimited, depending on list size and services offered.
- Paid quarterly in arrears on basis of claims.

Pros

- Rewards GPs providing a range of services with high uptake, e.g. vaccinations and smears, minor surgery.
- Money not limited by competing demands locally.
- Explicit conditions laid out in Red Book.

Cons

- Record keeping/claiming adds to administration burden.
- A disincentive to work in deprived areas with mobile populations, the homeless and refugees who will affect target payments.
- Targets such as large bonuses for hitting 90% vaccination targets create a potential conflict of interest, e.g. in vaccination advice, and may lead to conscientious objectors being removed from lists to protect payments.
- Cost-time disincentive for treating certain patient groups, e.g. homeless.
- Does not reward innovation.
- Limited career choices for GPs, e.g. some may not want to be principals or buy in.
- Perpetuates the status quo, by paying GPs in affluent areas well for providing high smear uptakes etc. rather than those who need them most, i.e. in deprived areas.

PMS Contract

Key Points

- Locally negotiated according to local needs and priorities.
- Provides more flexible employment options, e.g. salaried posts.
- Aims to reduce bureaucracy; payments made annually.

Pros

- Allows projects to be developed in areas of need, e.g. homeless clinics, which would not have been financially viable otherwise.
- Even cash flow throughout year.
- Allows locally appropriate targets to be set, e.g. areas with high elderly lists might prioritise monthly medication reviews rather than MMR uptake.
- May allow GPs to take over management of local facilities, e.g. community hospitals.
- Extra funding for manpower in early contracts, may reduce workload.
- Encourages innovative practices, e.g. nurse practitioner minor illness clinics.
- Provides for alternative methods of funding practice accommodation.

Cons

- Cash limited by local resources, e.g. if cottage hospitals overspend savings may have to be made from GP budget.
- Danger that new conditions may be unilaterally imposed, e.g. 48-hour access targets.
- Social injustice of offering bribes to those that sign up early on, rather than universally.
- Verification of services required, so administration savings may be illusory.
- No national bargaining, so in talks may be coerced into contracts by PCT.
- Creating new posts of salaried GPs may further exacerbate the shortage of applicants for principal posts.

Proposed Updated GMS Contract

Key Points

- Nationally negotiated, may not be changed unilaterally.
- Funded centrally.
- National targets.
- Graded incentive payments to encourage improvements in quality.
- End of mandatory 24 hour responsibility for patients.
- Provides a career structure designed to meet changing needs and aspirations through career.

Pros

- Encourages GPs to develop and maintain special interests.
- Promotes quality, e.g. Quality Practice Award.
- Should ease retention problems through better career development.
- Aims to reduce individual workload and should increase consultation times.

Cons

- Not yet costed.
- Several areas of debate unresolved, e.g. pensions.
- Potential to exacerbate quality/deprivation divide, with big well-run affluent practices reaching top quality targets easily, getting more funds, while deprived areas do not.
- If substantial numbers of GPs give up 24 hour responsibility, who will do the out-of-hours work? NHS Direct?

Paper 3

Answer 1   See reference material 3.1a, an extract from 'Survival outcome of care by specialist surgeons in breast cancer: a study of 3786 patients in the west of Scotland' (reprinted with copyright permission from *British Medical Journal* 1996; 312: 145–148).

Comment on the design of the study

- The study is a retrospective cohort study, and includes all the patients treated in the west of Scotland over the study period. This form of study is appropriate for comparing outcome between two groups. These were identified from the cancer registry and confirmed histologically, which should give universal coverage with minimal selection bias.
- Classification of surgeons as specialists by one person on the basis of local perception is extremely subjective and introduces a powerful source of bias.
- Follow-up was at least 5 years from diagnosis, making the results comparable with the standard index of mortality, the 5 year survival rate.
- The analysis of the data took account of other potential confounders such as tumour size, age, socio-economic status and nodal involvement. It did not take into account co-morbidity, which may be a confounder.
- The outcome measures included 10 year mortality, but follow-up only continued up to 1993, 5 years after the last cohort was recruited. This may allow reporting bias to influence results, with patients dying after the end of the study but within 10 years of diagnosis not being included.

Comment on the results in table 1 (reference material 3.1b)

- The results suggest that there is a statistically significant difference in survival between specialist surgeons and non-specialist surgeons.
- This difference persists when age, deprivation, nodes and tumour size are accounted for.
- The confidence intervals for all of these favour the results, suggesting they are true.

Give possible alternative explanations

- Specialist surgeons may give better treatment, and may refer more appropriately for adjuvant treatment, resulting in better survival rates.
- The study does not account for tumour type e.g. ductal carcinoma in situ vs fungating tumour, which may affect the results.
- Similarly, no account is made of the use of adjuvant treatment, e.g. tamoxifen, chemotherapy or radiotherapy, which are more likely to be

available in large specialist hospitals.
- Non-specialists are more likely to work in hospitals with small patient numbers and it has been shown that patient volume affects outcomes.
- The west of Scotland is a diverse area with many remote communities distant from the centres of excellence. Patients with advanced disease or other medical problems may not be referred or may decline referral to these centres on grounds of distance or transport difficulties. These may not be detected by deprivation scores.
- The use of lymph node involvement in the analysis relies on lymph nodes being sampled. This is more likely to be done by specialist surgeons.

Answer 2   A concerned father brings his 14-year-old son asking you to screen him for drugs. Discuss the issues this raises.

Drug misuse is an increasing problem amongst teenagers with risks not only to health but having implications for education, family relationships and crime.

Doctor Issues

- Responsibility to father and son. Need good rapport and address needs of both.
- Be non-judgmental/advocate for both. Assure confidentiality.
- Possibly long, difficult consultation. Best to see both father and son individually and together. Both may be angry; try to defuse tension.
- Be aware of your own feelings. Consider debriefing with colleagues over a cup of tea afterwards.
- May identify lack of knowledge on issues of consent, drug misuse or efficacy of testing.
- May feel out of depth and prefer to refer to local drugs service/paediatrician.
- Consider asking medical defence society for advice.

Patient Issues

For the Father

- Why attend today? Is son in trouble with police or school, or unwell?
- What are his ideas about drug use? Is he or other family member using drugs?
- What does he know about drug screening? Needs to understand implications for son, i.e. illegal activity may affect employment prospects.
- Need to inform him about issues of consent, i.e. son's autonomy and right to refuse testing under Children Act. Parents do not have automatic right to override.

For the Son

- Need to assess competence – can refuse to consent if understands purpose of procedure, and consequence of the results.

- If using, may not see as a problem especially if 'soft' drugs e.g. cannabis. May need education.
- Assess knowledge of risks of drug misuse, e.g. HIV/hepatitis if injecting. Consider examination. Opportunity for health promotion.
- Assess for psychological problems (e.g. depression) and problems at home or school (e.g. bullying or abuse).
- May resent father's interference – try to help him understand father's concerns.
- May be pleased at opportunity to seek help, e.g. may not had courage to admit it previously.
- Advise about availability for help, e.g. local drugs service, helplines, teenage psychiatric services.

Practice Issues

- Is surgery adolescent friendly? Are there leaflets/posters on related topics and where to seek help?
- Are all staff (e.g. nurses) aware of issues of confidentiality and consent?
- Are staff up-to-date on signs of drug abuse and local management options?
- Drug abusers can be aggressive – are safety procedures in place?
- Does practice have treatment policy? One GP seeing all drug abusers or refer all to drugs service?

Local Issues

- What services available in area to help drug abusers? Adequate provision and funding?
- Education may need outreach by drug workers to schools/youth groups.
- Involve local media in campaigns on risks and where to seek help.

National/Society Issues

- Need to address situations that cause drug abuse – deprivation, lack of activities for youngsters.
- Media portrayal of drug use may glamorise it.
- Experimentation is part of adolescence so need adequate education for both children and parents of the risks.
- Should responsibility for preventing drug abuse rest on the NHS rather than parents and schools?
- As society do we need open debate or more liberal policies on 'soft' drugs, as in the Netherlands?
- Drug treatment services and advertising campaigns need more resources.
- Need to tackle drug smuggling and dealing to reduce availability on streets.

Answer 3   A 33-year-old man asks to be referred for a circumcision, informing you this was suggested after a consultation over the internet for premature ejaculation. Outline your management of this consultation.

Sexual problems are common, often involving an underlying psychological or psychosexual reason. This patient has taken time to seek solutions to his problem on the internet, showing his concern about his symptoms. The consultation may be difficult for both doctor and patient.

Approach to Consultation

- Attain rapport by listening to the patient's request, encouraging him through open questions. Acknowledge his possible embarrassment, and the importance of the problem to him.
- GP may feel embarrassed, irritated, or threatened by patient seeking advice from the internet.
- Are you comfortable with taking a sexual history and the treatment options?
- Avoid presumptions about sexuality.
- Take a full sexual history, avoid jargon and use the patient's own terms.
- What does he mean by premature ejaculation? How long has the problem been going on?
- Explore psychosexual situation. Any underlying psychological difficulties? New partner? Is the relationship threatened by the problem? Any other stressors at home or at work?
- Has he already tried other methods of treatment?
- Explore ideas, concerns and expectations. Any other reason for his request, e.g. does his partner wish him to be circumcised? Are there religious reasons?
- Offer to read the internet information.
- Be honest if you are unfamiliar with circumcision as a treatment for premature ejaculation.
- As patient's advocate, explain need to assess the information for bias, poor research or potential risks.
- Examination: If indicated from history, and offer a chaperone if needed.
- Summarise his concerns and expectations. Agree a management plan with him putting this in the context of the request.
- Offering a joint consultation with his partner may be helpful and might identify psychosexual problems. Are they concerned about the premature ejaculation?
- Discuss other treatment options which include stop/start technique, books such as *Treat Yourself To Sex*.
- If necessary consider referral for psychosexual therapy (e.g. to Relate), family planning or a private counsellor rather than a referral to a urologist.

Ethical Issues

- Non-malificence: Avoid harm by what may be an inappropriate referral for an operation. Explain the potential for bogus advice on the internet. Explain possible detrimental health effects.
- Benificence: Avoid belittling the patient's request and involve him in the management plan.

- Autonomy: For the patient – respect his request and acknowledge his efforts in seeking a solution to his problem; for the doctor – ability to decide on treatment or management plan.
- Confidentiality: explain you will not discuss the problem with his partner without his consent.

Wider Issues

- Internet information
  – Pros: Potential for increased availability of information. Many sites e.g. patient support groups, Royal Colleges, or charities are good quality, allowing patients to learn about their diagnosis and be well informed in consultations.
  – Cons: Unfiltered information, may be biased, poorly researched or suggest treatments which can be purchased directly bypassing usual doctor.
- Medicolegal considerations: questions over where responsibility lies for internet consultations that may be in other countries.
- Any learning needs?
  – Well man clinics may allow opportunity to discuss sexual health issues with the doctor or practice nurse in a more informal clinic setting.
  – Are there any patient information leaflets on sexual problems which could be made available within the practice?

Answer 4 A hostel for the homeless is to be opened in your practice area. With reference to the literature, comment on the following areas of care for these patients, under the headings Factors and Comments and Evidence:

Factors	Comments and Evidence
Barriers to care **Patient factors** Registration	• Low registration reduces continuity of care and preventative care: only 24% of rough sleepers registered with GPs (1, 2). • Most care through accident and emergency departments (3).
Alienation	• Statutory agencies ill-designed to meet problems, often provoking inadequate responses to homeless people. Hospitals and GPs are reluctant to take them on, benefits regulations penalise them, council housing departments are interested only in families and the most vulnerable, and the police may move them on or arrest them for drunkenness.
Priorities	• Physical and psychiatric care are low priorities for homeless people. Food, shelter and money are more pressing than appointments with doctors or nurses. Low rates of prescription redemption (43%) may reflect this (4).

Factors	Comments and Evidence
Professional factors	
Professional attitudes:	
Stereotyping	• Homeless people seen as alcoholics with personality disorders, who choose their lifestyle.
Nihilism	• Doctors' usual interventions assume social factors (housing, adequate nutrition, and a social network) that make health and treatment possible. Many feel the absence of these defeats any medical or psychiatric intervention.
Organisation of services	• Mentally ill homeless people need multi-agency help – health, social, housing, psychiatric care. Requires close liaison which is the exception rather than the norm.
	• Many in primary care lack training and experience in homelessness.
	• Time-cost disincentive for GPs under GMS.
	• Philosophies of care: Some agencies operate policies that prevent or delay referral. Housing organisations assume tenants are responsible for behaviour and may evict if difficult patients deemed to have made a choice.
Medical problems	• 52% of homeless children and women have experienced physical abuse, in a Birmingham study (5).
	• Chronic chest, skin, and dental problems common and may exacerbate anxiety and depression.
	• London Coroner's records show that life expectancy was 42 years for rough sleepers (2).
	• *British Medical Journal* 1994 prevalence of schizophrenia in residents of hostels for the homeless 9% (6).
	• Homelessness may be a cause or a consequence of mental health problems.
	• Homeless children are significantly more likely to have delayed development, learning difficulties, and higher rates of mental health problems. These often persist after rehousing (6).
	• Poor compliance with treatment and frequent drug and alcohol misuse may exacerbate problems (1).
Provision of care	• PMS removes time-cost disincentive through salaried posts, but PMS practices risk becoming ghettoes for the homeless, rather than integrating them in mainstream healthcare. They should be a bridge, addressing immediate needs then facilitating reintegration. PCTs ideally placed for this role, and ideal role for nurse practitioners (2).

References

1. ABC of mental health: Mental health on the margins. *British Medical Journal* 1997; 315: 536–539
2. Developments in the provision of primary health care for homeless people. *British Journal of General Practice* Feb 2002
3. Use of hospital services by homeless families in an inner London health district. *British Medical Journal* 1989; 299(6701): 725–727
4. Homeless people miss out on prescribed treatment. *British Medical Journal* 1994; 308: 135
5. Mental health problems of homeless children and families: longitudinal study. *British Medical Journal* 1998; 316: 899–902
6. Comparison of prevalence of schizophrenia among residents of hostels for homeless people in 1966 and 1992. *British Medical Journal* 1994; 308: 816–819

Answer 5   A 15-year-old girl complains of problems 'down below'. What issues surround this consultation?

This embarrassing problem has a number of causes and is a potentially difficult consultation. Good rapport and sensitivity are vital.

Factors to Consider

- For a male doctor, is she happy to see you? May want a female GP or nurse.
- May need female chaperone, especially for examination.
- She is a minor. Do you feel happy to see her alone? Are parents aware she is attending?
- Need to ensure she is competent to consent to questioning or examination. If concerns about possible abuse, consider advice from paediatricians.
- Assure of confidentiality unless suspected abuse or rape. Her safety is paramount and you may be obliged to notify social services or police in this situation.
- Do you feel comfortable discussing sex with a 15 year old girl? You may be embarrassed, or have strong views on underage sex especially if you have teenage daughters. Do not allow feelings to affect consultation.
- What is your knowledge of vaginal discharge; if not confident, family planning/GUM clinic referral. May highlight learning need.

History

- Establish her concerns. Is she worried about STDs, pregnancy, gynaecological disease e.g. cancer or infertility? Has a friend or family member recently developed any of these?
- How long has discharge been present? Discuss nature of discharge, any bleeding, abdominal pain or itch? Has she had it before? Recent antibiotics or steroids causing candida?
- Is she sexually active? Contraception or condoms? LMP, establish risk of pregnancy.

- Does a partner have symptoms?
- Is her agenda contraceptive advice or seeking advice about STDs? Is she 'Gillick' competent?
- Consider if she could be in a non-concensual sexual relationship – rape or abuse. If partner is older, having sex with minor illegal even if she consents.
- Does she have psychological illness, e.g. depression, causing preoccupation with health?

Examination

- Consider vulval/speculum examination to take HVS/chlamydial swabs and look for signs of abuse.
- Consider pregnancy test.
- General examination, e.g. for signs of diabetes, eczema.

Management

- Offer treatment depending on likely cause.
- Consider stat treatments for increased compliance, e.g. azithromycin.
- Discuss sexual health. Provide details of GUM/family planning clinic for further advice. Give leaflets.
- Discuss contraception and encourage to return.

Issues for Practice

- How teenage friendly is practice? Need easy access to appointments with choice of medical staff, posters and leaflets about sexual health, contraception. Emphasise confidentiality.
- Need easy access to chaperones for male GPs.
- Consider outreach to schools or youth groups to educate about services available and sexual health.
- Co-ordinate efforts with school nurses.

Local Issues

- Teenagers important target group for funding.
- May need to improve access to services e.g. teenage walk-in clinics outside school hours.
- Use local media to highlight issues on sexual health and how to seek help.

National Issues

- Health of Nation/Sexual Health and HIV policies target sexual health and teenage pregnancy rates.
- Ensure adequate sex education in schools.
- Try to remove some of taboos on discussing sex openly in society.
- National campaigns e.g. to screen for chlamydia, advocate safe sex, etc.
- Funding for sexual health advice and contraception, e.g. more family planning and GUM clinics.

Answer 6   A 48-year-old woman asks for a repeat thyroxine script, started recently for weight loss by one of your partners. Her BMI is 26 and no thyroid blood tests are recorded. How do you manage this request?

This puts the doctor in an awkward position, as there appears to be no clear clinical indication for the prescription. This request raises a number of issues.

Ethical Considerations

- Autonomy: we reserve the right to act according to our principles, including not to prescribe.
- Non-malificence: do not cause harm by unsafe prescribing.
- Benificence: not prescribing avoids risk to physical health but harm may arise from loss of trust in her doctor or from feeling a treatment is being withheld.

Consultation Considerations

- Need for tact and a non-confrontational style. Patient expecting a repeat script may be alarmed if questioned in detail.
- Establish the facts. Is this a safe prescription request?
- Who commenced the treatment? Care needed to avoid loss of trust in the doctor–patient relationship.
- Why was prescription started?
- Have any tests been done that are not recorded in the notes?
- What does she understand about her treatment and the reasons for commencing thyroxine?
- Was script requested by the patient, e.g. after hearing of people losing weight this way?
- Review previous attempts at weight loss, e.g. diet/exercise/weight watchers.
- Explore her health beliefs regarding weight loss.
- Any cautions or contraindications for thyroxine use, e.g. ischaemic heart disease.
- Any side effects of treatment, e.g. angina, palpitations or dyspnoea.
- Examine patient to check for signs of hypothyroidism or hyperthyroidism.

Management Options

Immediate

- If unable to prescribe, explain why but respect her relationship with her usual GP. Explain that different doctors often manage clinical situations in different ways.
- Suggest she see your partner to discuss the prescription.
- Review notes looking for diagnosis of hypothyroidism or thyroxine treatment.
- Suggest alternative weight loss management e.g. practice nurse clinic.
- Risks to doctor–patient relationship of refusal may warrant a limited script

after explaining risks.
- Importance of good records.

Future

- Discuss with the GP in a non-confrontational way, e.g. 'I noticed Mrs . . . was on thyroxine but I wasn't quite sure why . . .', allowing her GP to explain the prescription.
- Was this on specialist advice and has there been inadequate documentation?
- Has the doctor recently read an article that suggests the treatment?
- Has the doctor felt pressurised to prescribe to end a difficult consultation or to please the patient?
- Discuss at practice prescribing or significant event meeting.
- If the partner is unrepentant, you may need to contact LMC/GMC. You have a duty to act if colleagues are unsafe.

Practice Issues

- Potential conflict between the partners; handle with care. Avoid jumping to conclusions.
- Clinical governance. Audit of other patients on thyroxine and weight loss management. Is this a one-off, or one of many?
- Is it a problem of inadequate record keeping or aberrant prescribing?
- Does it identify learning needs for the doctor involved?
- Anticipate the possibility of a complaint.

Wider Issues

- No national guidelines on obesity management support the routine use of thyroxine. Specialist clinics may prescribe thyroxine under close supervision, and this difference in medical practice and opinion can lead to conflicts.
- Medico-legal aspects. Risk of serious side effects e.g. AF or chest pain occur on inappropriately prescribed treatment. Contact medical defence organisation.
- Local PCO/CHImp may become involved if found to be a widespread prescribing issue.

Answer 7   *What are the difficulties in dealing with doctors as patients?*

Ethical Issues

- Confidentiality: Remain professional and keep consultations within the surgery. Avoid temptation of continuing consultations in a social setting.
- Justice/equality: Should treat as any other patient.
- Autonomy: Doctor may feel under pressure to pursue clinical course at variance with own diagnosis. Need to acknowledge patient's ideas and expectations about a particular course of action.

Consultation Issues

- Doctor's feelings. May find it a difficult consultation. May feel under scrutiny or apprehension/ego boost that colleague is coming to consult.
- Time-keeping. May be stressed or embarrassed if running late? Effect on previous/subsequent patients if try to catch up prior to the consult or if over-run.
- Aim for patient-centred approach, get to the bottom of concerns and expectations.
- Need to share clinical findings and clinical diagnosis and agree management plan.
- Professional status, e.g. seniority. The patient may be more knowledgeable or experienced with the problem presented. Should they be referred to another partner or specialist?

Patient Issues

- Often unregistered, and consulting GP may not have their old medical records.
- May expect to be treated differently, e.g. invited into the reception office rather than waiting in the waiting room.
- Frequently self-medicate before consultation, clouding the clinical picture or delay diagnosis.
- They may also be treating other family members or attending out of courtesy but expecting a referral on to a specialist.
- Psychological /relationship/drug/alcohol issues. High incidence of all these in the medical profession. Embarrassment may prevent attendance.
- Patient's feelings. May have inaccurate health beliefs, e.g. a consultant psychiatrist thinking he has bowel cancer when he has piles, and have unrealistic expectations of treatment/referral.

Practice Issues

- Should the GPs within a practice register with another practice to avoid conflicts of interest?
- Preferential treatment, e.g. may expect to be put straight through to GP to discuss case/investigations, or to be given contact number for out of hours.
- Costs – more likely to request expensive medication or investigations (which may be unnecessary).
- Higher referral rate to outpatients for second opinions or treatment.
- Is there a policy relating to notes for staff/professional colleagues? Notes need to be secure, e.g. by blocking access via security levels on computers or locking hand-held notes in a separate area.

Answer 8   You are a member of a working party carrying out a review of community care of patients with Parkinson's disease. You are keen to make any decisions evidence-based.

Outline how you would gather your evidence

- The evidence should be gathered by first deciding on a research question, e.g. 'Are community nurses effective in preventing hospital admissions in Parkinson's disease.'
- The next stage is to agree a search strategy, e.g. all medical and nursing journals published in English.
- Searches are made of databases (e.g. Medline, Cochrane Collaboration) and local resources (e.g. medical library).
- Supplementary information can be gained from asking interested parties, e.g. local neurologist.
- Once the search is complete, the results should be screened. The screening process should be agreed by stakeholders to avoid bias and be hierarchical, e.g. first preference for systematic reviews, then randomised controlled trials, down to case reports.
- The screening should also take into account relevance of location, e.g. UK studies more relevant to UK practice, quality of journal (is it peer reviewed?) and quality of research.

Comment on the strengths and weaknesses of the study design, intervention and sampling methods (reference material 3.2a)

Strengths

- Set in UK primary care, with practices selected at random in nine health authority areas each also selected at random from all over England, making the data more likely to be applicable in general.
- All practices in the selected areas were invited to participate, reducing risks of inclusion bias. Exclusion criteria were minimal, which improves generalisability.
- The length of the study and the number of participants was sufficient to detect any genuine effects, and a sample size was calculated to ensure power.
- Nurses received standardised training and resource package and had standardised responsibilities.
- Assessment of outcomes was by trained lay interviewers with standardised tools. This would reduce bias.
- Outcome measures were clear and objective.

Weaknesses

- It is unclear whether the study was limited to Parkinson's disease or all patients with parkinsonism.
- It is not possible to tell where the areas studied are. They may be scattered all over the UK, giving a heterogeneous population representative of the country, or they may be clustered in a small area.
- The control group received no extra help of any description. It may be that the process of someone visiting is beneficial, rather than any specific nursing intervention, and this may bias the quality of life assessment.
- The nursing time use study was only done over two 1-week periods.

These periods may not be representative of the 2-year period and the nurse may alter her working pattern in the knowledge that she is being observed.

- The intervention is difficult to quantify through time use study. There is no objective recording of what the nurses were actually doing, e.g. telephone calls could be to arrange physiotherapy or could be to cancel the newspapers for a patient.

Answer 9   Extracts from the results of the paper entitled 'Effects of community based nurses specializing in Parkinson's disease on health outcomes and costs: randomized controlled trial' (reprinted with copyright permission from *British Medical Journal* 2002, 324; 1072–1075) are given in reference material 3.3a.

How do the results support a decision in favour of the intervention?

The subjective change in general health between the groups was significantly better in the intervention group.

How do the presented results support a decision against the intervention?

- There was no significant difference between the intervention and control groups in severity of disease, mortality or fractures.
- No differences were observed in the objective measures of wellbeing.
- The only statistically significant improvement was not a primary outcome and it is unclear when this was included. This may be a source of bias.

Comment on the analysis of the costs

- Cost analysis shows that the intervention group were more expensive than the control group, but this includes the cost of the nurses. When this is allowed for the costs are almost equal. A breakdown of the costs shows that institutional costs, primary care and drug costs were lower for the intervention group. These results suggest that although the overall costs may be the same, the money may be being spent differently, e.g. increased home help costs allowing patients to stay at home rather than going into institutions.

Are there any other explanations for the lack of effect in the results?

- The nurses were newly trained. They may have been on a steep learning curve, spending much of their time learning local systems and increasing their expertise.
- The nurses spent much of their time in administrative tasks and driving. It may be that if they concentrated more on clinical interventions they would have been more effective.
- No standardised diagnosis of Parkinson's disease. Relying on GP records may bring in patients with other conditions misdiagnosed with Parkinson's, e.g. essential tremor, although if these were evenly distributed between control and intervention groups they would make less impact.

Answer 10   You see a 55-year-old woman who works in a pottery with her husband. She tells you she has been seen at the walk-in centre, who told her that she should be referred to the allergy clinic regarding a rash. What issues does this raise, and how would you proceed?

This problem raises several difficult issues and requires a considered approach to produce a mutually acceptable result.

Consultation Issues

- Preconceived agenda. Need to acknowledge concerns and expectations and be open to negotiation.
- Take account of her husband. He may require a different style of consultation.
- Difficult consultations often over-run and this may have adverse effects on the GP. May need to agree to deal with some issues today, leaving others for later.

Patient Issues

- Why does she want a referral? Have her previous consultations been unrewarding?
- What are her ideas, concerns and expectations? Does she think the rash is occupational? Is she hoping for compensation or to retire on medical grounds due to an occupational condition?
- Why did she go to the walk-in centre rather than the GP as a first step?
- Is she trying to play off the walk-in centre against the GP? Has she been refused a referral in the past?
- What would be the gain of a referral for her? Confirmation of allergy, allowing allergen avoidance?
- What are drawbacks of a referral? If the tests are negative how would she feel? What would she do?
- Are there any other problems in her life, e.g. marital difficulties or desperation to leave her job?

Doctor Issues

- Acknowledge own feelings, e.g. irritation at demanding patients or walk-in centre which may prejudice approach to the patient.
- Conflict of interest between role as patient's advocate and gatekeeper for secondary care
- Acknowledge own limitations in allergy and occupational medicine, and be prepared to refer if beyond these limitations.
- Any learning need?

Issues for Society

- Walk-in centres. Do the public find second opinions independent of their GP helpful or confusing?
- Should nurses with computers be advising patients to ask for secondary care referrals? Do they just allow patients to manipulate the system,

playing GPs off against the walk-in centre and vice versa?
- Is the benefits system a disincentive to work?

Management of Problem

- Acknowledge problem and review history. Definite pattern of allergy? What treatments have been tried? Is it purely occupational or does it occur at home? Can she take steps to avoid exposure at work?
- Examine patient. Is the rash typically allergic? Any evidence of other cause, e.g. SLE?
- Explain diagnosis in simple terms. Explain therapeutic options, e.g. start with non-sedating antihistamines, gloves, barrier or steroid creams. Offer trial of treatment for one month and refer if no better.
- Explain role of allergy testing, including chance of negative results. Acknowledge that proven allergy may suggest an occupational component, but explain implications, e.g. need to change jobs.
- Agree a mutually acceptable management plan, e.g. trial of non-sedating antihistamine for 1 month and refer if no better.
- Offer early consultation to review or reinforce information.
- Review call report from walk-in centre. Was the outcome as reported? Is there a problem with walk-in centre advice? Consider feedback, either positive or negative.
- Ideally recharge before next patient, e.g. with a cup of tea if at all possible.
- If you feel the consultation has gone badly, discuss with partners or Balint group.

Answer 11 Osteoporosis is a significant problem. For each of the three parts to the question, write your answers in separate columns under the headings Factors and Comments and Evidence:

Factors	Comments and Evidence
Prevention of osteoporosis	
Identifying those at risk	Royal College of Physicians guidelines (1) suggest risk factors should be sought: previous fragility fracture, untreated hypogonadism, glucocorticoids >7.5 mg prednisolone a day >6 months, disease associated with osteoporosis e.g. hyperthyroidism, radiological osteopenia, family history and low BMI.
Lifestyle measures	*British Medical Journal* review (2) suggests not smoking, regular weight-bearing exercise and adequate diet are protective. A meta-analysis in *British Medical Journal* 1997 (3) suggested 1 in 8 hip fractures in women attributed to smoking.
Drugs for prevention	• HRT and SERMs (e.g. raloxifene) preserve bone mass (4) and can be used in those at high risk. Raloxifene has no effect on the breast.

Factors	Comments and Evidence
	• Some evidence that statins may reduce fracture risk (5). • National Osteoporosis Society guidelines for the treatment of steroid-induced osteoporosis suggest treatment with bisphosphonates prophylactically if dose over 15 mg/day.

Prevention of fracture

Systematic review confirmed benefits of exercise classes, occupational therapy input, hip protectors and medication reviews to avoid iatrogenic falls (6). Balance training reduces falls by 30%.

Investigation

RCP guidelines suggest FBC, LFT, ESR, TFT, bone studies as baseline, with further tests as appropriate, e.g. FSH if hypogonadism suspected. DEXA scan confirms presence of osteoporosis. Consider testing vitamin D levels (7).

Treatment

• In established osteoporosis, calcium, vitamin D (8) and bisphosphonates (9) have been shown to prevent fractures.
• HRT prevents fractures but needs to be taken long term (10).
• Parathyroid hormone injections have been shown to increase bone mass (11) and reduce fractures by 90%.

References

1. *Osteoporosis – clinical guidelines for prevention and treatment.* Royal College of Physicians.
2. Recent advances in rheumatology. *British Medical Journal* 2000; 321: 882–885
3. A meta-analysis of cigarette smoking, bone mineral density and risk of hip fracture: recognition of a major effect. *BMJ* 1997; 315: 841–846
4. Preventing osteoporosis, falls, and fractures among elderly people. *British Medical Journal* 1999; 318: 205–206
5. Raloxifene to prevent postmenopausal osteoporosis. *Drug and Therapeutics Bulletin* 1999; 37(5): 33–36.
6. HMG-CoA reductase inhibitors and the risk of fractures. *JAMA* 2000; 283(24): 3205–3210
7. Editorial – Managing osteoporosis in older people with fractures. *British Medical Journal* 1999; 318 (7182): 477
8. Effect of calcium and vitamin D supplementation on bone density in men and women of 65years and older. *New England Journal of Medicine* 1997; 337: 670–676
9. Treatment with aledronate prevents fractures in women at highest risk. Results from the Fracture Intervention Trial. *Archives of Internal Medicine* 1997; 157: 2617–2624
10. HRT and fracture risk *Bandolier* 2002; 96: 4–5

11. Effect of parathyroid hormone (1–34) on fractures and bone mineral density in postmenopausal women with osteoporosis. *New England Journal of Medicine* 2001; 344: 1434

Answer 12   For each of the following scenarios, comment on the treatments and give evidence to support your views.

A 76-year-old man with Parkinson's disease

- A 5-year comparison of levodopa and ropinirole found less dyskinesia in ropinirole group but no difference in functional abilities (1). Ropinirole seemed to be better tolerated, but there was 50% drop out in both groups. The authors concluded that early Parkinson's disease can be managed successfully for up to 5 years with a reduced risk of dyskinesia by initiating treatment with ropinirole alone and supplementing it with levodopa if necessary.
- Clinical evidence (2) suggests selegiline may be of benefit, but one study suggests increased mortality. Dopamine agonists better for younger patients.
- Depressive and anxiety disorders affect at least half of patients with Parkinson's disease but are under-recognised and inadequately treated. Treatment may improve global condition, and SSRIs may be beneficial in these patients (3).
- Physiotherapy may have a small effect on mobility, but costs are high and benefits small (4).
- Potential long-term benefits from pallidotomy, with less dyskinesia and tremor, but no long-term improvement in functional abilities (5).

A 29-year-old woman with PMS

- Vitamin B6 shows effective for depressive and physical symptoms at dosage of 50 mg twice daily (6).
- Clinical evidence (7) suggests NSAIDs and SSRIs are beneficial, chiropractic and evening primrose oil likely to be beneficial.
- A systematic review concluded that SSRIs are an effective first-line therapy for severe PMS with acceptable side effects and safety (7,8).
- Systematic review concludes no evidence for efficacy of progestogens (9).
- Vitex agnus castus effective and safe (10).
- Some evidence that Yasmin, a COCP containing a spironolactone-like progestogen, is beneficial in severe PMS. Conflicting evidence for the benefit of other COCP's (11).

A 74-year-old man with benign prostatic hypertrophy

The choice of treatments is (12):

- Watch and wait.
- Finasteride blocks androgens; may cause impotence, gynaecomastia or osteoporosis. PLESS study found less symptoms, retention and need for surgery. Takes weeks to work, so less suitable for obstructive symptoms. May mask cancer by reducing PSA.

- Alpha blockers, uroselective (e.g. tamsulosin) or non-selective, reduce bladder tone. May cause postural hypotension, although less of a problem with uroselective drugs. May be more effective than finasteride (13). The efficacy of tyrazosin, finasteride, or both in benign prostatic hyperplasia.
- Surgery: Best reserved for severe symptoms as high incidence of side effects.

Guidelines suggest:

- Mild symptoms: Watch and wait.
- Moderate symptoms: Start with uroselective alpha blocker, then finasteride if ineffective.
- Severe symptoms: Refer.

References

1. A five-year study of the incidence of dyskinesia in patients with early Parkinson's disease who were treated with ropinirole or levodopa. *New England Journal of Medicine* 2000; 342:1484–1491
2. What are the effects of drug treatments in people with early Parkinson's disease? *Clinical Evidence* 7 (August 2002) Section: Neurological Disorders, Parkinson's Disease
3. Editorial – Treatment of early Parkinson's disease. *British Medical Journal* 2000; 321: 1–2
4. MS, Parkinson's disease and physiotherapy. *Drug and Therapeutics Bulletin* 2002; 40: 38–40
5. Long-term follow-up of unilateral pallidotomy in advanced Parkinson's disease. *New England Journal of Medicine* 2000: 342; 1708–1714
6. Efficacy of vitamin B_6 in the treatment of premenstrual syndrome: systematic review. *British Medical Journal* 1999; 318: 1375–1381
7. Effects of treatments for women with premenstrual syndrome *Clinical Evidence* 7 (August 2002) Section: Women's Health, Premenstrual Syndrome
8. Efficacy of selective serotonin reuptake inhibitors in premenstrual syndrome: a systematic review. *The Lancet* 2000; 356: 1131–1136
9. Efficacy of progesterone and progestogens in management of premenstrual syndrome: systematic review. *British Medical Journal* 2001; 323: 77
10. Treatment for the premenstrual syndrome with agnus castus fruit extract: prospective, randomised, placebo controlled study. *British Medical Journal* 2001; 322: 134–137
11. Evaluation of a unique oral contraceptive in the treatment of premenstrual dysphoric disorder. *J Womens Health Gend Based Med* 2001 10(6): 561–569
12. Benign prostatic hyperplasia. *British Medical Journal* 1999; 318: 343–344
13. The efficacy of terazosin, finasteride, or both in benign prostatic hyperplasia. *New England Journal of Medicine* 1996 vol 335: 533–540

Paper 4

Answer 1 You see a 31-year-old man who has a purulent urethral discharge. Outline your management.

Consultation Style

- Potentially awkward consultation. Aim to be open, honest and non-judgmental.
- Compliance and follow-up critical and depend on patient feeling understood and supported.
- Questions should be unambiguous and simple. Avoid assumptions about sexuality.
- Avoid own feelings and prejudices, e.g. about promiscuity affecting consultation.
- Offer GUM referral, with benefits of greater confidentiality and rapid on the spot diagnosis and better able to perform contact tracing.

History

- Take a full sexual history, including previous history of infections.
- How was infection acquired?
- Any associated symptoms, e.g. dysuria, conjunctivitis, joint pain?
- Any special risks, e.g. sex with a prostitute, or in sub-Saharan Africa?
- Is he at risk of HIV?
- Explore health belief model. Understanding of STDs, treatment and follow up?

Examination

- Examine genitalia. Urethral swabs for chlamydia and standard culture. Consider rectal and throat swabs if any anal or oral sex. Evidence of other STDs, e.g. inguinal lymph nodes (lymphogranuloma venereum), ulcers (syphilis or herpes)?
- General examination for signs of other disease, e.g. hepatitis, or lymphadenopathy if HIV is a possibility.

Contact Tracing

- Emphasise need for open and honest discussion with sexual contacts
- Need for screening and treatment of partner to prevent reinfection of patient, infection of others or untreated disease in contacts.

Treatment

- If compliance likely to be poor, consider stat doses, e.g. azithromycin.

- If gonorrhoea likely give ciprofloxacin. Co-infection with chlamydia common so have a low threshold for treating after taking swabs.
- Advice on safe sex and give condoms if appropriate. Advice on risk of reinfection if partner not treated.

Summarise

- Explain likely diagnosis and implications.
- Offer opportunity to ask questions. How do they feel about diagnosis? Do they acknowledge the diagnosis? Any preconceptions, e.g. I cannot get gonorrhoea because I have only had sex once in last year with my boyfriend. Only homosexuals get AIDS, etc.
- Explain treatment and procedure for results of swabs sent.
- Arrange follow-up for results, and to discuss further tests e.g. HIV, hepatitis.
- Offer written information about the issues covered, and give information about GUM clinic.

Practice Issues

- Check confidentiality policy regarding sensitive results, e.g. not to be given over phone, etc.
- Need for more health information regarding STDs, e.g. posters in waiting room?
- Is there a learning need for the GP/nurses, e.g. current guidelines for treatment?
- Is there a problem with access to GUM services? Consider raising with PCT.
- Acknowledge own feelings after consultation, perhaps have a cup of tea before the next patient.

Answer 2

You are telephoned by the daughter of Mr Smith, an 81-year-old widower who lives alone. She lives in Canada and visits infrequently. She says that he is unsafe living alone and wants you to put him into a home. What issues does this raise?

This potentially difficult problem requires a sensitive, cautious approach, acknowledging the feelings and wishes of all involved.

Issues Relating to the Consultation

- Difficulties of telephone consultations, with lack of visual cues and pressures of cost of overseas calls.
- Be aware that daughter lives in country with a different healthcare system, where services and attitudes to autonomy may be different. This may require patient explanation; you should not assume that the daughter understands the UK system.

Issues Relating to the Daughter

- You risk breaching Mr Smith's confidentiality in discussions with daughter. Even though she may be next of kin he still has the right to confidentiality. Explain that you can record her concerns and act on them but are unable to give medical details without consent.

- Ideas, concerns and expectations: What are her concerns? Any new symptoms that you were unaware of, e.g. falls? Is she aware of risky behaviour, e.g. heavy drinking? Have neighbours expressed concerns to her? What does she expect?
- Why has she telephoned now? Does she feel guilty because she is not caring for him?
- Any other motive for wanting him put in a home, e.g. the sale of his property?
- Does she have enduring power of attorney over his affairs? If so, she may be able to make decisions for him.

Issues Relating to Mr Smith

- Autonomy: Is he mentally competent? If so, he has the right to self-determination and removing him from his house would be an infringement of his human rights.
- Risk: Is he at risk, e.g. of falling, drinking too much. Is he able to look after himself?
- Is he depressed or lonely? Has daughter picked this up, triggering her call?
- Has there been a change in his medical condition, e.g. heart failure that has rendered him bed-bound?
- Is he getting any help at home from family locally or social services?

Issues for the GP

- Acknowledge daughter's concerns. It is easy to become irritated with absent relatives who make apparently unreasonable demands.
- Be prepared to reassess his medical, psychological and social situation, and act accordingly.
- Review record keeping, e.g. regarding next of kin, power of attorney, at-risk register for elderly?

Implications for the PHCT

- If Mr Smith is genuinely at risk, why has this not been picked up before?
- Does the practice need to be proactive in care of elderly, e.g. health visitor to carry out over-75 checks?
- Is there a problem with social services resources in the area?
- Any learning needs regarding rights of patients and relatives in this situation?

Answer 3   A 14-year-old boy comes to see you with his parents. He has just been discharged from hospital after having an epileptic seizure. What issues would you aim to cover and what would be your management aims?

This situation raises a number of issues both for the patient and his family, and for the practice. The aims of management are to minimise seizures and achieve a normal quality of life.

Consultation Issues

- Do not hurry. Encourage everyone to contribute. Solicit his views particularly, without talking over him.
- Encourage them to take notes if they wish.
- Explore their beliefs about epilepsy, and accommodate these.
- Bear in mind they may be going through a form of bereavement.
- Investigate their ideas, concerns and expectations? Do they blame themselves, e.g. for dropping him as a baby? Are they terrified it is genetic, and thus avoid future pregnancies? Do they fear he will be mentally handicapped?
- What are his ideas, concerns and expectations? Driving, choice of career?

Medical Issues

- Review history, including current working diagnosis. What have they been told?
- What future investigations are planned and what follow up?
- Review treatment: Is he being treated at present?
- Are they aware of side effects of treatment, e.g. need to check blood levels? Drug interactions?
- Do they know what to do in event of another seizure?
- Agree treatment goals: Aim for minimal seizures, normal quality of life.
- Explain that if seizure free on medication he may be able to stop his drugs and drive later.

Health and Safety Issues

- Explain need to avoid potentially dangerous sports, e.g. swimming alone.
- Advise the family re provoking factors, and avoidance.
- Is there a need to educate school, e.g. what he can and cannot do?

Social Issues

- Encourage him to be open with friends and family about his problem. Surveys suggest >50% do not even tell their fiancées.
- Explain need to comply with medication and anticipate problems, e.g. with drinking, dancing, etc.
- Give written advice about support groups e.g. British Epilepsy Association.

Practice Issues

- Does the practice need to audit its care of people with epilepsy? Surveys suggest GP care is often substandard.
- Is there a need for a register, with appropriate follow-up, drug monitoring, ensuring compliance and identification of side effects?
- Any learning needs?

Answer 4   You practice in a busy urban practice with high deprivation scores. One of your partners announces at the practice meeting that he wants to become a trainer. What are the implications of his request?

This situation may arise for a number of reasons and affects the practice at many levels.

Implications for the partner who wishes to become a trainer

- Why does he want to be a trainer? Does he no longer find work fulfilling? Is this escapism?
- May enhance clinical skills and knowledge through teaching.
- Will need to go on trainers' course, resulting in time away from surgery and will lose 1–2 sessions a week through tutorials and joint surgeries when training.
- May find interruptions to surgery to help trainee disruptive and stressful.
- Will have burden of supervision and paperwork in addition to normal workload.
- Must be prepared to be challenged by trainee.

Implications for the Practice

- Need to provide a room and secretarial time for trainee.
- Need to be aware of trainee's requirements (e.g. video consent forms), and be able to advise patients about the trainee and what they do.
- Practice facilities may need upgrading, e.g. installation of video camera.
- Staff need to know limitations of trainee, not to consider them as another partner.
- Need to ensure protected time for trainee, may need assistance with audit, etc.
- Will need adequate notices to inform patients, including practice leaflet.

Implications for Partners

- Individual workload may be higher at first, due to loss of trainer's sessions and slow pace of a new trainee, but lower later.
- Trainee may need supervision when trainer is away.
- May be concern about trainees being present at practice meetings
- Need to clarify situation regarding out-of-hours care, to avoid resentment over who the trainee does sessions for.
- Some financial benefit as trainee's salary paid by health authority and training grant payable to practice.
- Trainee more likely to make mistakes; partners need to be aware of this and compensate accordingly
- Need ground rules regarding trainee, e.g. working unsupervised, particularly early on.

Implications for Patients

- May lack confidence in trainee's skills/advice, or relish the opportunity for a fresh opinion.
- May be popular with certain patients, e.g. young women if the trainee is a woman.
- May be asked to participate in video surgeries. May not feel able to say no.
- May be concerned about confidentiality, particularly in video surgeries.
- May find joint surgeries awkward.
- May not understand difference between a medical student and a trainee.
- May abuse the trainee, e.g. for drug seeking or sick certification.
- Trainees often run behind, causing agitation for patients.

Answer 5   Discuss the usefulness of the following in the diagnosis and management of eating disorders. Give evidence to support your views:

Diagnostic tools

- The SCOFF questionnaire (1) has high sensitivity and specificity with low false positive rate, and is acceptable and memorable:
    - Do you make yourself **Sick** because you feel uncomfortably full?
    - Do you worry you have lost **Control** over how much you eat?
    - Have you recently lost more than **One** stone in a 3 month period?
    - Do you believe yourself to be **Fat** when others say you are too thin?
    - Would you say that **Food** dominates your life?

    One point for every 'yes'; a score of 2 indicates a likely case of anorexia nervosa or bulimia.

- Diagnosis improved if look for common character traits, e.g. shyness, natural insecurity, alexithymia (2).
- DSM IV criteria should be used if in doubt.
- Wide variations in recognition and referral of eating disorders in general practice (3).

Cognitive behavioural therapy (CBT)

- Some evidence for the efficacy of psychotherapy and CBT but the studies were limited, e.g. not blinded (4).
- CBT was likely to be beneficial both on its own and in combination with antidepressants, although again the studies were limited e.g. blinding, different outcomes, etc. (5)
- Formal CBT is more effective than self-directed psychological techniques with a manual, but self-directed therapy may be useful where access is limited (6).

Drug therapy

- SSRIs can reduce bulimic symptoms in the short term, but there is

insufficient evidence of long-term efficacy (5).
- Tricyclics tend to cause weight gain, hence may exacerbate symptoms.
- There is also some evidence from meta-analysis that combination therapy of CBT plus SSRI is better than SSRI alone (7).

References

1. The SCOFF questionnaire: assessment of a new screening tool for eating disorders. *British Medical Journal* 1999; 319: 1467–1468
2. Eating disordered patients: personality, alexithymia, and implications for primary health care. *British Journal of General Practice* 2000; 450: 21
3. Eating disorder service: GP referral to: why the wide variation? *British Journal of General Practice* 2000; 50: 380–383
4. *Cochrane Database Systematic Review* 2000; 4: CD000562.
5. *Clinical Evidence* 2001
6. First step in managing bulimia nervosa: controlled trial of therapeutic manual *British Medical Journal* 1994; 308: 686–689
7. Combination of antidepressants and psychotherapy for bulimia nervosa: a systematic review. *Acta Psychiatrica Scandinavica* 2000; 101: 256–264

Answer 6   What are the difficulties when dealing with patients who abuse opiate drugs?

The DOH sees primary care as the ideal setting for treatment of drug abuse. There are a number of potential problems in caring for these patients.

Problems for the Patient

- Does the patient know how to contact the doctor and use the appointment system?
- Chaotic lifestyle may cause difficulties in attending for appointments.
- Prejudice: Attitudes of previous doctors and reception staff (e.g. removal from list) may alienate or impede rapport.
- Social circumstances: Lack of support or family guidance can hinder healthcare. Drugs users are more likely to be unemployed, have a history of crime and live in poor housing. May be malnourished.
- Drug users are less likely to be offered preventative healthcare by the practice, and less likely to take it up.

Problems During the Consultation

- Rapport: Engage the patient and allow respect for autonomy. Avoid adopting a parental role. Involve the patient in decisions.
- You may be biased by past experiences with drug abusers or perceive pressure to prescribe. Address problems at face value. Addicts often present in a crisis or with complex or difficult requests.
- Safety. Consider a position near the door if there is a risk of violence. Is there a panic alarm?
- Consider a treatment plan or contract with the patient. This needs to be

explicit and agreed early, e.g. not attending when drunk/under influence of drugs, always to see same doctor.

- Make explicit rules if you agree to prescribe drugs, e.g. no lost scripts/early scripts.
- Social issues: are the 'at risk' children or partner. Are there any court cases pending?
- Seek mental health or other medical problems, e.g. sepsis, heart murmurs.
- Consider contacting previous doctor/drugs services for previous history. Shared care, e.g. with drugs services, can lead to the problems of manipulation or repetition.
- Is there a need for urinary screening for drugs?

Problems for the Practice

- Practice policy: Practices sometimes refuse all intravenous drug abusers as regular patients, in which case they need to be directed to an appropriate source of medical care.
- Consider a named doctor always to see patient for continuity of care and to avoid manipulation. May need to ensure patients see a partner rather than the registrar or locum.
- Prescribing policy: Do the doctors prescribe methadone? If so, is this under the support or guidance of the local specialist drug team? Risks of prescribing in patients who still inject.
- Contracts: The receptionists need to know which patients are being seen under 'contract' and what the contract entails, e.g. only to see a particular doctor.
- Staff safety: All staff need to know about violent patients. Mark notes as high risk, or put alert message on the computer.
- Staff concerns and prejudice: Allow staff to express concerns at meetings and formulate solutions.
- HIV/hepatitis risk: Consider marking notes as high risk. Ideally the patient should be informed.
- Notification of addicts is encouraged by the DOH.
- Workload implications: May attract other drug abusers. The average addict undergoing treatment has been shown to consult up to 32 times per year.
- Funding: If large numbers of addicts approach PCT for funding. Possible PMS contract.
- Security: Consider risks of prescription fraud, etc.

Ethical Considerations

- Justice: All patients should be treated fairly with respect to medical care.
- Autonomy: Patient's right to choose lifestyle. GP's right to autonomy on prescribing decisions.
- Benificence: Avoid inflicting harm or failing to prevent harm, e.g. not providing necessary care.
- Non-maleficence: Offer choices in their care and to minimise risk of

harm, e.g. prescribing methadone inappropriately.

Answer 7   Outline ways in which practices can improve access for the disabled.

We have a moral and legal duty to ensure practices provide adequate access for the disabled, and this may take several forms.

Assess Current Situation

- Consider the skill base within the practice staff, e.g. lip reading.
- Consider the range of disabilities likely to be encountered now and in the future, e.g. physical, intellectual, impaired hearing, vision or speech.
- What facilities already exist?
- Involve all the staff for a broad perspective on problems and possible improvements.
- Does the practice leaflet include access for the disabled? Is it clear and suitable, e.g. Braille?
- Audit access. Disabled parking? Wide doorways and disabled toilets? Wheelchair ramps or lifts if consulting upstairs?

Premises Improvements

- Consider outreach clinics e.g. local schools for the disabled, with doctor seeing patients in familiar surroundings or scheduled visits to local nursing homes.
- Clearly visible signs, e.g. large font.
- Consider Braille on important signs and notices within the surgery.
- If there is a call system, can patients hear or see it? Consider an induction loop for hearing aids.
- Privacy for hard of hearing: is there a soundproofed area for giving results or talking to receptionist?

Improving Staff Skills

- Staff training should include appreciation of problems experienced by disabled patients.
- Respect for autonomy, patience and sensitivity are essential when dealing with patients.
- Doctor–patient relationship enhanced if patient feels their problems are understood.
- Consider the patient's mental capacity. Can they understand appointment times?

Other Issues

- Clarify the carer's position and role – mental advocate or assistant with mobility? Carer's register should be established. What are their needs?
- Patient's autonomy should be respected and patient involved in decisions where possible.
- Consider patient's confidentiality, establish whether they wish the carer

to be present and what information may be shared with them.
* Patients group should involve disabled representatives.
* Any useful ideas from other practices?
* Look at links and involvement of social services, financially and for practical support.
* Is there any funding available from the local primary care organization?

Answer 8   **Mr Smith consults you with symptoms of atrial fibrillation. What evidence is there to help you decide on the value of the following aspects of care?**

Control of rate

MeReC Bulletin March 2002 (1):
* Digoxin best for sedentary patients with persistent atrial fibrillation (AF). Less effective if high sympathetic drive, e.g. hyperthyroidism. Inotropic, so good if heart failure. Does not cardiovert. May prolong attacks of paroxysmal AF. Narrow therapeutic range. Toxic in renal impairment or hypokalaemia.
* Beta blocker or rate-limiting calcium antagonist (verapamil or diltiazem) more suitable for IHD or hypertensives and hyperthyroidism. Avoid calcium antagonists in heart failure.
* Danger of bradycardia if verapamil used with beta blocker.

Reducing risk of thromboembolism

MeReC Bulletin March 2002 (1):
* All patients including paroxysmal AF should be considered for aspirin or warfarin.
* Choice based on risk of stroke vs risk of bleeding:
Risk of stroke (TIA/CVE)
Very high – Warfarin
High (>65 y.o., BP, DM, LV dysfunction, heart failure) – Warfarin
Moderate (>65 y.o. or <65 y.o. + other risk as above) – Aspirin or warfarin
Low (<65 y.o., no risk factors) – Little benefit from either
* Prospective study of stroke prevention found warfarin underused in practice (2).
* Stroke Prevention in Atrial Fibrillation (SPAF) (3) supports warfarin, but this study was secondary care-based with strict exclusion criteria. Absolute risk of haemorrhage 1.3% p.a, number needed to harm 60.

Aspirin or warfarin?

* A systematic review found no significant difference between aspirin and warfarin in fatal CVE and borderline difference in non-fatal CVE (4).
* Primary care-based study in lone AF >60 y.o. found no difference in favourable or unfavourable outcomes, but these patients are low risk (5).
* Near patient INR testing shown to be effective in managing

anticoagulation (6).
- Patient information about risks and benefits of anticoagulation, followed by patient choice regarding treatment, showed 40% declined warfarin (7).

Control of rhythm

MeReC Bulletin March 2002 (1):
- Cardioversion if AF <48 h duration (low risk of thromboembolism), especially if compromised.
- Anticoagulate first if duration over 48 h.
- Amiodarone safest drug in heart failure to maintain sinus rhythm. Potential side effects on liver and thyroid; check LFT/TFT 6 monthly.

References

1. *MeReC Bulletin* March 2002
2. Kalra et al. Prospective cohort study to determine if trial efficacy of anticoagulation for stroke prevention in atrial fibrillation translates into clinical effectiveness. *British Medical Journal* 2000; 320: 1236–1239
3. Stroke Prevention in Atrial Fibrillation (SPAF) Investigators. Stroke prevention in atrial fibrillation study, final results. *Circulation* 1991; 84: 527–39
4. Systematic review of long term anticoagulation or antiplatelet treatment in patients with non-rheumatic atrial fibrillation. *British Medical Journal* 2001; 322: 321–326
5. Primary prevention of arterial thromboembolism in non-rheumatic atrial fibrillation in primary care: randomised controlled trial comparing two intensities of coumarin with aspirin. *British Medical Journal* 1999; 319: 958–964
6. Oral anticoagulation self-management and management by a specialist anticoagulation clinic: a randomised cross-over comparison. *Lancet* 2000; 356: 97–102
7. The impact of patients' preferences on the treatment of atrial fibrillation: observational study of patient based decision analysis. *British Medical Journal* 2000; 320: 1380–1384

Answer 9   Mr Jones, who has complained of impotence since being treated for a heart attack, asks for a prescription for sildenafil (Viagra), which you have not previously prescribed. You agree to look into it and come across an article entitled 'Systematic review of randomized controlled trials of sildenafil (Viagra) in the treatment of male erectile dysfunction' (reprinted with permission by *British Journal of General Practice* 2001; 51: 1004–1011; reference material 4.1).

Comment on the selection process used

- The researchers sought to identify all published and unpublished randomised controlled trials. The electronic and hand searches were

thorough, together with further searches of references in the identified papers. This should identify all relevant published trials.
- The description is not specific as to how unpublished trials were sought. It may be that Pfizer have omitted to provide unpublished trials showing lack of effect, i.e. inclusion bias towards trials showing effect.
- Assessment of quality was undertaken by two independent researchers. This should help to minimise inclusion bias.

Comment on the studies identified

- The search identified 20 trials with 4000 participants, including a broad range of aetiologies such as spinal cord damage, diabetes and idiopathic erectile dysfunction. This large number, together with the long follow-up of 6 months, should give an adequate sample population.
- Exclusion criteria were broad with a lot of exclusions which may limit the generalisability of the study to a general practice population.
- Data on withdrawals was not reported, which is unfortunate since the side effect profile is clinically relevant, but analysis was done on an intention-to-treat basis.

Comment on the endpoints used

The endpoints were clinically relevant, and used a standardised system. Secondary endpoints were also included for some studies such as quality of life questionnaires and partner questionnaires, which gives an indication of overall acceptability.

Comment on the results in Fig.1 and their applicability to Mr Jones

- These studies all show a statistically significant effect of sildenafil in the Global Efficacy question 'Did treatment improve your erections?' The confidence intervals for individual studies are all in the positive zone favouring treatment, and the Forest plot shows that the combined results give a risk difference of 0.537 with narrow confidence intervals of 0.484–0.589). This suggests a NNT of 2.
- Mr Jones has IHD and thus would have been excluded from these studies. For this reason it is not possible to extrapolate these data regarding safety or efficacy to him.

Answer 10   Statins: a panacea for all ills? Comment, with reference to current evidence.

Statins have been shown to be beneficial in many parts of the body. Their effectiveness can be considered in the following areas

Cardiac Effects

Primary Prevention of Ischaemic Heart Disease

- Meta-analysis showed a reduction of 30% in cardiac events (1).
- WOSCOPS showed benefit of treating asymptomatic men with high cholesterol levels (2).

- AFCAPS/TexCAPS study showed benefits of treating asymptomatic men and women with normal cholesterol to prevent cardiac events (3).

Secondary Prevention of Ischaemic Heart Disease

- 4S study: relative risk reduction of 30% in statin users with previously high cholesterol (4).
- CARE study showed benefits in secondary prevention for people with normal cholesterol (5).
- Heart Protection Study (6): 5 years of statins typically prevents heart attacks, strokes, or other major vascular events in:
  – 1 in 10 people who have had a heart attack
  – 8 in 100 people with angina or some other signs of coronary heart disease
  – 7 in 100 people who have ever had a stroke
  – 7 in 100 people with diabetes.

Effects on Bone

Evidence from the UK General Practice Research Database suggests statins reduce fracture rates (7).

Effects on CNS

Stroke

Systematic review supports use of statins in people with prior stroke, coronary heart disease, and a cholesterol concentration >5mmol/l (or low density lipoprotein cholesterol concentration >3mmol/l) (8).

Alzheimer's

Statins are associated with a 79% reduction in the risk of Alzheimer's disease (9).

Macular Degeneration

A cross-sectional study suggests patients on statins have significantly lower rates of macular degeneration (10).

Other Effects

There is some evidence that statins may be useful in preventing transplant rejection (11).

Problems with Statin Use

- Many people fail to get full benefit due to lack of access (i.e. they are not offered statins) (12).
- Intolerable side effects, with discontinuation rates up to 30% in one study (13) May cause myositis, liver enzyme abnormalities and GI side effects as well as interfering with sleep.

References

1. Use of lipid lowering drugs for primary prevention of coronary heart disease: meta-analysis of randomised trials. *British Medical Journal* 2000; 321: 983

2. Prevention of coronary heart disease with pravastatin in men with hypercholesterolemia. *New England Journal of Medicine* 1995; 333: 1301–1307

3. Primary prevention of acute coronary events with lovastatin in men and women with average cholesterol levels. Results of AFCAPS/TexCAPS. *JAMA* 1998; 279: 1615–1622

4. Scandinavian Simvastatin Survival Study Group. Randomised trial of cholesterol lowering in 4444 patient with coronary heart disease: the Scandinavian Simvastatin Survival Study (4S). *Lancet* 1994; 344: 1383–1389

5. The effect of pravastatin on coronary events after myocardial infarction in patients with average cholesterol levels. *New England Journal of Medicine* 1996; 335: 1001–1009

6. Statins are the new aspirin. *British Medical Journal* 2001; 323: 1145

7. HMG-CoA reductase inhibitors and the risk of fractures. *JAMA* 2000; 283(24): 3205–3210

8. Cholesterol lowering with statin drugs, risk of stroke, and total mortality. An overview of randomised trials. *JAMA* 1997; 278(4): 313–321

9. Study adds to evidence that statins reduce risk of Alzheimer's disease *British Medical Journal* 2002; 324: 936

10. Risk of macular degeneration in users of statins: cross sectional study. *British Medical Journal* 2001; 323: 375–376

11. Statins as a newly recognized type of immunomodulator *Nature Medicine* 2000; 6: 1399–1402

12. Editorial – Statins: underused by those who would benefit. *British Medical Journal* 2000; 321: 971–972

13. Discontinuation rates for use of statins are high. *British Medical Journal* 2000; 321: 1084

Answer 11   Your practice is looking at designing a protocol for the management of blood pressure in the nurse-led diabetic clinic. You wish the process to be evidence-based. See reference material 4.2a, an extract from the paper 'Tight blood pressure control and risk of macrovascular and microvascular complications in type 2 diabetes:UK PDS 38' (with permission from *British Medical Journal* 1998; 317: 703–713)

Comment on the strengths and weaknesses of the methodology

- The study had a focused research question: to determine whether tight control reduced complications.
- The population were recruited from general practice but managed in

hospital outpatients, which may reduce generalisability to primary care.
- The inclusion criteria included fasting plasma glucose >6 mmol/l on two consecutive mornings. This is lower than the WHO diagnostic criteria and may have resulted in misdiagnosis of normal patients or those with impaired glucose tolerance rather than type 2 diabetes.
- Patients who could not take beta blockers (i.e. could not safely be randomised), or those who had a requirement for strict blood pressure control were excluded. These are reasonable exclusion criteria since it would be unethical to randomise patients to less strict control that might harm them.
- Randomisation produced baseline characteristics that were essentially similar in every respect except for visual acuity which was significantly worse in the less tight treatment group. The ethnic mix was the same, which is important as different ethnic groups respond differently to certain drugs.
- The treatment protocol used a target BP of 200/105 but this was reduced half way through the trial. This may bias the results in favour of tight control, since damage may have been done in terms of complications before the change to lower limits.

Comment on the results shown in Fig. 4

- There is a statistically significant reduction in any diabetes-related endpoint, deaths related to diabetes, microvascular complications and stroke, all with p values <0.05.
- The confidence intervals are wide, however, and approach the line of no effect.
- The absolute risk reductions are 16% for all endpoints, 6% for deaths related to diabetes, 7% for microvascular disease and 5% for stroke.
- This represents numbers needed to treat of 6, 16, 16 and 20 to prevent each of these endpoints.

Comment on the overall validity of the results

- Studies of ACE inhibitors have shown that these have a beneficial effect on vasculature independent of their antihypertensive properties. The system of allocating patients to either tight control with ACE inhibitors or loose control without, may mean that it is not the tight blood pressure control but the ACE inhibitor that is responsible.
- Comparing tight control with any drug combination to loose control with any drug combination would have answered this question.
- In particular, the finding that stroke is less common in the tight control group may be due to this effect, since the HOPE study has shown that stroke is reduced in patients on ramipril despite a mean blood pressure reduction of only 3/2 mmHg.
- The endpoints for retinal photocoagulation are potentially subjective and this combined with the difference in visual acuities between the two groups may have introduced bias.

- The baseline characteristics in terms of treatment of diabetes are given at randomization, but not at the end of the trial. Patients within the tight control group could have had different treatments for diabetes e.g. higher use of insulin, which may have been confounding.

Comment on the generalisability of the results to general practice

- The patients were not all diabetic on conventional WHO criteria, since the cut-off used was fasting plasma glucose of 6 mmol/l, so the results may not be applicable to care of all diabetics.
- Follow-up was done in the hospital outpatient setting which may bring better blood pressure control than GP based treatment. Similarly, there may be an exaggerated 'white coat' hypertension response at hospital compared with GP, giving even tighter control as a result.

Answer 12 Your practice is attempting to shorten access times to comply with government targets. One of the areas you decide to concentrate on is frequent attenders. See reference material 4.3a, an extract from 'Psychosocial, lifestyle, and health status variables in predicting high attendance among adults' (with permission from *British Journal of General Practice* 2001; 51: 987–994).

Comment on the strengths and weaknesses of the methodology

Strengths

- Clear aims, study design appropriate in attempting to answer the question.
- Study carried out in metropolitan UK, covering all practices within a 30-mile radius of the administrative centre. This makes it less prone to inclusion bias.
- The postal questionnaire method gives a good cross-sectional coverage, but relies on good records from GPs of up-to-date addresses.
- The questionnaire used validated indices to get objective assessments of various factors, allowing comparison between different groups.
- The sample size was calculated before the study, and the number of participants exceeded the calculation, which should give the study sufficient power.
- The statistical analysis was specified in the paper and is a validated method.
- Respondents were compared with national statistics to test whether they are representative of the country as a whole.
- The questionnaire responses were validated by comparing self-reported attendance with medical records for a sample of patients.

Weaknesses

- The administrative centre is not specified; it may be in the area of

Southampton around the university with socio-demographic characteristics not typical of the city as a whole. Within that area there were only six general practices. This suggests either low population density or large multidoctor practices. These may not be representative of inner city or rural practices.
- Written questionnaires are less likely to be filled out by those whose first language is not English, who are illiterate or who have visual problems. All of these are potentially high users of services.
- Using a postal questionnaire together with information leaflets for another study may lead participants to feel they are being criticised about their attendance, and those with high attendances may not respond. It might have been better to use the questionnaire on all patients attending surgery.
- Not including those over 80 or in nursing homes, and children, removes a large percentage of frequent attenders. Information on these patients is important in analysing workload.

Comment on the results given in Table 2 and Table 4 of reference material 4.3b

- These show statistically significant associations with female sex and no academic qualifications (p values 0.006 and <0.001 respectively).
- None of the other associations in Table 2 are statistically significant.
- In Table 4 there are statistically significant associations with medically unexplained symptoms (p = 0.006), health anxiety (p = 0.001), perceived health (p < 0.001), lack of negative attitudes to doctors (p < 0.001) and not trying the pharmacist first (p < 0.001). Low alcohol use is associated with attendance (p = 0.002).

Suggest possible interventions based on these results

- Measures to try and combat health anxiety and perceived health, e.g. CBT, may be appropriate in reducing attendance.
- Tackling medically unexplained symptoms is difficult and therapies such as CBT may be more expensive in terms of resources and time than the savings to be made in reduced attendance.
- Encouraging more use of the pharmacist may not be effective if the people who attend the doctor first have psychological or complex needs that cannot be addressed by a consultation with a pharmacist. Transferring large quantities of work to pharmacists may result in them charging for this service, negating any savings made.

Paper 5

Answer 1   A local headmaster with type 2 diabetes refuses to take medication, preferring homeopathic treatment. He refuses to attend the diabetic clinic. Bloods show a fasting blood sugar of 12, HbA1c 9.6, BP 184/102, BMI 36. How would you manage his care?

This situation requires tact and patience to ensure a mutually acceptable outcome. The GP should aim to have an open consulting style that actively solicits and acknowledges the patient's thoughts and feelings. He is a professional man and will expect to be treated accordingly.

Review History

- Explain diagnosis, relate to any symptoms he may have.
- Explore health beliefs: knowledge of diabetes, treatment and complications?
- Worried that he will have to give up driving if he admits he is diabetic?
- Worried that he may lose his job and income? Terrified of injections?
- Explore feelings about diagnosis. Does he believe he has diabetes? Try to answer his questions. Does he fear stigma of chronic disease?
- Any family history of note, e.g. ischaemic heart disease?
- Any confounding factors, e.g. steroids giving false positive results?
- Discuss events since diagnosis. Did he refuse to attend the nurse-led clinic because of denial, inconvenient timing or because he did not want to be seen by a nurse? Genuine belief in alternative medicine or denial?
- Does he accept diagnosis? Did he have unacceptable drug side effects e.g. diarrohea from metformin, leading him to homeopathy?

Examination and Investigations

- Examine for complications and co-morbidity. Test urine for protein and blood pressure (nephropathy), visual acuity, BMI, evidence of neuropathy.
- Arrange ECG. Check fasting lipids.

Explain the Findings

- Explain diagnosis and presence and relevance of any complications. Give realistic prognosis. Aim of treatment is normal quality of life and a normal life expectancy (St Vincent Declaration).
- Explain planned treatment and importance of lifestyle (healthy diet, exercise, smoking and ideal weight).
- Explain how the practice manages diabetes. Offer choice of nurse-led clinic or GP. Importance of retinal screening.

- Explain the implications of diagnosis. He must inform DVLA and car insurers. Eligible for free prescriptions, if on drug therapy.
- Give written information, including the British Diabetic Association.

Agree Treatment Goals and Plan Treatment

- Realistic goals. Start with lifestyle, i.e diet, exercise. Consider dietician referral.
- Aim for monthly reviews at convenient time if possible. Offer early review or telephone advice.
- Promote nurse-led clinic. Evidence suggests better routine care.
- If he fails to respond, he will need drug treatment, ideally with metformin initially, together with control of his blood pressure (UK PDS study).
- If there are complications, consider referral to an endocrinologist.
- Consider writing to homeopath to ensure care is complementary rather than antagonistic.
- Ensure the patient is on the diabetes register
- Consider initial hospital referral for advice/reinforcement of message.

Review Case at Next PHCT Meeting

- Do patients have a problem attending diabetic clinic?
- Is everyone consistent in their diagnosis of diabetes? Does everyone know the latest diagnostic criteria?
- Any learning needs, e.g. when to use insulin?
- Are many patients turning to complementary medicine? If so, does this reflect a problem with the service patients are getting?

Answer 2   Following an audit by the GP registrar it has been brought to your attention as trainer that one of the senior partners has been prescribing excessive amounts of benzodiazepines. What issues are raised by this?

Frequent prescribing of benzodiazepines is discouraged because of problems of addiction, tolerance, withdrawal and risk of falls in the elderly.

Issues Relating to the Audit

- Why was it done? After a significant event?
- Was this issue already known to be a problem within the practice and an audit performed by a temporary member of staff such as the GP registrar seen as a good way of bringing it into the open?
- Who initiated the audit – the registrar, or a partner/trainer?
- Danger of audit being seen as an underhand way of investigating one person's practice.
- Was everyone in the practice aware that an audit was taking place?
- How was the audit conducted – across the practice or only involving certain partners? Was the methodology used accurate and the conclusions drawn appropriate?

Issues for the Registrar

- The topic of the audit and the results obtained could cause difficulties for the partner identified. They could feel like a scapegoat.
- Are they uncomfortable about bringing such information into the open?
- How does it effect their relationship with the partner concerned? May result in interpersonal difficulties or avoidance.
- May effect interactions with other practice staff, e.g. may not trust the registrar.
- May worry about future job prospects if widely known to be a 'trouble maker'.

Issues for the Trainer

- Responsible to the practice patients and staff but also for the well-being and support of registrar.
- The situation may represent a conflict of interest.
- Need to deal appropriately with the information putting the safety of patients first (following GMC guidelines) but also deal sensitively with the partner concerned.
- Consider involving practice manager, possible meeting in private with partner concerned to discuss audit and look for causes.
- Should the results of the audit be presented anonymously or be completely open? Who should attend? Partners and practice manager or other staff?
- Agree rules, e.g. significant event type session without blame.
- Consider seeking advice from LMC/protection societies.

Issues for the Senior Partner

- Why is he prescribing so much? May be legitimate, e.g. lots of psychiatric patients, drug users or patients withdrawing from alcohol.
- Prescriptions could have been initiated by specialists or by a previous doctor, i.e. patients on this medication for many years and unable or not prepared to stop.
- Does this identify a need for education? E.g. of risks of benzodiazepines and alternatives available, or methods of treating addiction and services available to help.
- Other areas of his practice might also be dangerous. Does he need a full review of practice/re-education?
- Could this be prescription fraud with illegal selling of benzodiazepines?
- Could he have medical problems, e.g. alcohol/drug misuse, and be self-medicating? This audit may be the catalyst needed for him to admit the problem and seek help.
- Is this a reflection of burnout? Easier to just give benzodiazepine script rather than explore and deal with problems.
- If addicted or under stress may need advice on BMA/LMC counselling services or support group for addicted physicians.

Issues for the Practice

- If there are concerns over this doctor's fitness to practice, you should consider reporting him to the GMC.
- If criminal activity is suspected, you may need to involve the police.
- There may be legal implications, e.g. litigation against the practice for inappropriate prescribing.
- The audit may highlight issues about repeat prescribing policy. Is it computerised, allowing closer monitoring and audit? Are systems in place to prevent excessive repeats?
- Involve local pharmacy advisors to help improve prescribing.
- Consider tackling the problems of the patients on benzodiazepines.
- Consider re-audit after changes have been implemented.

Issues for Society

- Minimise prescription fraud – better monitoring and prevention strategies.
- Better services for drug addicts may reduce value of drugs such as benzodiazepines on the streets.
- This problem may eventually be detected by reappraisal/revalidation systems if missed by the practice.

Answer 3   A 40-year-old civil engineer comes to you having recently been diagnosed with retinitis pigmentosa (autosomal dominant). He has two teenage daughters. What factors affect this consultation?

Retinitis pigmentosa is an autosomal dominant condition leading to progressive loss of sight.

Issues for the Patient

- Devastating diagnosis. May show bereavement type reaction – denial, anger, distress.
- No curative treatment available – feeling of powerlessness.
- An independent professional man may find it difficult to ask for help or show vulnerability.
- He may have received limited information at secondary care level. Is he aware of other sufferers? Does a parent or other family member have condition? What are his ideas, concerns and expectations?
- If no family members are affected there may be a possibility of paternity disputes.

Implications

- Work: May eventually have to give up. Loss of independence/autonomy/ income, together with loss of profession, pride in skills, social standing. May need retraining. Possible retirement on disability.
- Family: Guilt/distress over family implications, e.g. income if cannot work, genetic risks e.g. concern about children/future pregnancies. May have effect on relationship with wife/sex life. Does he have a good

support network?

Issues for the Doctor

- Potentially a long and difficult consultation which may overrun.
- Need to listen, be sympathetic. Aim to develop good relationship for future, for long-term support.
- Assess needs at this stage – what does he want? Does he need more information on diagnosis?
- Is he seeking testing for daughters or advice on how to break news to family?
- How well do you know this patient? Does he have other medical problems? What are his coping mechanisms?
- Assess for serious psychological distress – depression, suicide risk, drug/alcohol abuse.
- Practical issues: may need period off work to allow to adjust to diagnosis. At some stage he will need to notify his employer and the DVLA. Consider advice from specialist/occupational health.
- Has implications for mortgage/insurance applications.
- Offer contacts e.g. RNIB, self-help groups, leaflets. Will need specialist input, e.g. ophthalmology, geneticist.
- Appreciate your own emotions: you may be similar in age, professional with children. Recognise need to offload/discuss with colleague/raise with peers at Young Principals group.
- Possible area of limited knowledge – may make you uncomfortable.
- Need to address any learning needs for future consultations.

Issues for Teenage Daughters

- They may inherit the condition. Frightening diagnosis.
- Are they patients of yours? Decision needed with family on when to inform them. They have a right to know.
- Are they competent to consent to testing?
- Implications for career choice, driving licence, having a family, life insurance.
- Consider referral to local genetics service who have experience in counselling family members and offering support. Can put them in touch with other affected families.

Issues for Spouse/Partner

- When to tell them: may not be ready yet. Respect confidentiality.
- Implications for partner: may have to become breadwinner, potential financial difficulties for family. Psychological impact of diagnosis and prospect of husband's and daughters' disability.
- May have to be carer.

Wider Issues

- Limited provision of geneticists. Increasing recognition of genetic contribution to disease. Needs more funding.

   • Often lack of knowledge in primary care about genetic conditions.
     Rapidly expanding area of medicine needing better training and
     dissemination of information to GPs.

Answer 4   Obesity is a common problem. Comment on the following, giving
               evidence to support your views:

The value of treating obesity

   • A prospective study of obese children found that over 50% became obese
     adults with a high risk of developing the metabolic syndrome
     (hypertension, dyslipidaemia and insulin resistance). Weight loss in
     childhood was protective against developing this syndrome (1).
   • Even in the absence of hypertension, hyperglycaemia or dyslipidaemia,
     obese men are at increased cardiovascular risk (2).
   • Weight loss associated with reduced risk of diabetes, reduced all cause
     mortality and improved lipid profiles (3).
   • Obesity seems to be a particular risk factor for diabetes in South Asians,
     and juvenile onset type 2 diabetes was reported for the first time in obese
     white teenagers in the UK in 2002 (4, 5).

Drug treatment

   • Systematic review showed modest benefits of orlistat when combined
     with low calorie diet (*Clinical Evidence* 2000) (6).
   • Sibutramine shown in randomised controlled trials to be effective in
     overweight patients. Effects not sustained on discontinuation.
   • To date 34 deaths reported worldwide as a result of sibutramine, which
     has been suspended in Italy.
   • Sibutramine Trial of Obesity Reduction and Maintenance (STORM).
     Together with diet may produce 5–7% weight loss. Significant rises in
     blood pressure common (7).
   • NICE recommend sibutramine used for no longer than 1 year.
   • Significant side effects in 27% of subjects on orlistat; strict licensing
     restrictions, and may interfere with vitamin uptake (8).

Surgical treatment

The Swedish Obese Subjects (SOS) compared surgical intervention versus
standard therapy in obese individuals (mean BMI 40 kg/m^2) Mean weight
loss was 28 kg (SD 15) in patients and 0·5 kg in controls (8,9).
Post-operative mortality was 0·22% (9).

Lifestyle measures

   • Diet together with lifestyle measures are as effective as diet with
     structured aerobic exercise, and more acceptable to patients.
     Furthermore, cardiovascular risk profiles were improved equally between
     the two (10).
   • Novel diets, e.g. milk only, produced superior weight loss (average 9.4kg
     at 16 weeks) to both conventional diets and reported rates for drug

therapy. Outpatient based, so may not be strictly applicable to primary care (11).
- Primary care-based study of very low calorie diets produced mean weight loss of 15kg over 12 months, but there were strict exclusion criteria; all patients had BMI > 30 and patient numbers were small (12).
- Actively teaching healthy eating in schools produced an increase in vegetable consumption but no other changes in either general health or health of overweight children. A similar intervention in Singapore with restrictions on foods sold in the canteen and special attention for obese children has reduced rates of obesity, although the social circumstances in Singapore may limit applicability (13).

References

1. Relation between obesity from childhood to adulthood and the metabolic syndrome: population based study. *British Medical Journal* 1998; 317: 319–320
2. Abdominal obesity and the 'hypertriglyceridaemic waist' phenotype. *British Medical Journal* 2001; 322: 687–689
3. Why and how should adults lose weight? *Drug and Therapeutics Bulletin* 1998; 36(12): 89–92
4. Type 2 diabetes in obese white children. *Archives of Diseases of Childhood* 2002; 86: 207–208
5. Early evidence of ethnic differences in cardiovascular risk: cross sectional comparison of British South Asian and white children. *British Medical Journal* 2002; 324: 635
6. Endocrine disorders, obesity. Drug treatment in adults. Orlistat *Clinical Evidence 7* (August 2002)
7. Effect of sibutramine on weight maintenance after weight loss: a randomised trial. *Lancet* 2000; 356 (9248): 2119
8. Drug treatment for obesity. *British Medical Journal* 2001 322: 1379–1380
9. Sjostrom et al. Reduction in incidence of diabetes, hypertension and lipid disturbances after intentional weight loss induced by surgery: the SOS intervention study. *Obesity Research* 1999; 7: 477–485
10. Effects of lifestyle activity vs structured aerobic exercise in obese women. *JAMA* 1999 281: 335–340
11. Randomised controlled trial of novel, simple, and well supervised weight reducing diets in outpatients. *British Medical Journal* 1998; 317: 1487–1489
12. Obesity wars: a pilot study of very low calorie diets in obese patients in general practice. *British Journal of General Practice* 1998; 48: 1251–125
13. School based intervention has reduced obesity in Singapore. *British Medical Journal* 2002; 324: 427
14. School based programmes on obesity. *British Medical Journal* 2001; 323: 1018–1019

Answer 5   How can burnout be avoided?

A recent BMA survey showed the effect of ever increasing demands on the profession, with more GPs electing to work reduced hours and opting for early retirement. Recognition of burnout and its causes is increasingly important in a career in primary care.

Factors in Oneself

- Balance between work and relaxation: engage in outside activities, avoid taking work home, use strategies to 'switch off'.
- Choose a post to best suit your personality and skills e.g. size of practice, workload, type of surgery (rural/urban).
- You need to get on with colleagues. Look at options to explore interests e.g. hospital posts (clinical assistants), PCT work.
- Consider provision in partnership agreement, e.g. sabbaticals
- Look after your own health: register with GP, avoid self-diagnosis or medication. Exercise regularly. Take care with alcohol/smoking/drug misuse.
- Inability to admit when under stress may exacerbate problems. Be honest with yourself and your partners.

Practical Methods

- Find confidant to share problems, e.g. difficult patients, complaints, terminally ill patients and practice problems.
- Find mentors from other practices, e.g. by reciprocal arrangement.
- Keep motivated by engaging in continuing education, try to learn new skills, keep up to date. Personal learning plans may make this more interactive and more enjoyable.
- Young Principals group or meeting colleagues provides support, socially and educationally.
- Be aware of resources available if problems develop, e.g. BMA counselling service, LMC support available, local educational supervisors.

Practice Considerations

- Encourage supportive practice environment – hold regular practice meetings and identify problems early.
- Non-critical discussions of practice, e.g. significant event monitoring.
- Flexibility in practice, e.g. support outside activities.
- Hold away-days or team building activities for all staff, to encourage cohesiveness. Stress-management courses are an option.
- Ensure all involved in decision-making – gives a sense of ownership.
- Recognise signs of stress early in colleagues – anger, depression, loss of motivation, time off work, signs of alcohol/drug abuse, clinical mistakes, increased complaints.
- Intervene early, e.g. a meeting to discuss concerns allowing early referral

for help/education. Offer options such as reducing hours, less out-of-hours, time off, less non-clinical work (but impact on other staff may cause resentment).

Local Issues

- Deprived or rural areas often have inadequate numbers of GPs, resulting in more work and difficulty recruiting. PMS contracts may help overcome this with salaried posts.
- Single-handed or rural GPs may feel isolated and find difficulty in taking time off or finding a locum.
- Financial support from PCG for practice away days, e.g. locum funding may help, especially for small practices. Consider 'locum insurance' to allow sick leave without guilt.
- Provision of good, well-organised and staffed out-of-hours service, with option of reducing commitment may help reduce stress, especially with drivers for security.

National Strategies

- Government initiatives to reduce work load and improve morale, e.g. reduction in paperwork, less frequent changes to practice.
- Delegation of clinical work to nurses and non-clinical work to others such as clerical staff.
- Increase GP numbers through increased number of medical students and making GP more attractive to young doctors. Better remuneration and more respect.
- Encourage culture of openness about mistakes in NHS with stress seen less as a sign of weakness. Mistakes should be admitted without fear of retribution. Care of self should be seen as important part of good practice.
- Better funding available for support services, e.g. occupational health services for GPs. Easier access to help at all stages of medical career.

Answer 6   How does the evidence contribute to the management of chest infections in primary care? Comment on the following.

Diagnosis

It is necessary to distinguish between simple upper respiratory tract infection and pneumonia. Evidence suggests GPs are not very good at this:

- In a survey of patients in primary care, only 25% had abnormal signs but 70% were given antibiotics (1).
- GPs diagnosed pathogen type (viral or bacterial) correctly only 50% of the time (2).
- British Thoracic Society guidelines 2001: suspect pneumonia in patients with fever, cough, sputum and/or pleuritic pain and usually with localising signs on examination.

Evidence suggests GPs often know antibiotics will be ineffective, but prescribe them anyway to meet patients real or perceived expectation.

- Patients often expect antibiotics and are more likely to re-attend if they don't get them, i.e. you need to address patient's ideas, concerns and expectations (3).

Treatment

- A systematic review found antibiotics to be no better than placebo in treating acute cough in adults. Furthermore, 19% of patients experienced side effects (4).
- Higher prescribing for all respiratory tract infections is associated with significantly fewer admissions with complications, but the overall effect is modest (5).

Who Should get Antibiotics?

A *British Journal of General Practice* editorial (6) suggested the following should be considered for antibiotics:

- Anyone in whom pneumonia is suspected
- Patients over 60 with co-existent disease, e.g. heart disease
- Patients with COPD (these patients frequently need steroids as well).

What are the Alternatives to Prescribing?

- A realistic prognosis at initial consultation may be useful in preventing re-attendance, usually with information on antibiotics in the form of written leaflets (7).
- A review of cough medicines available without prescription concluded that there was no good evidence for their effectiveness (8).
- Studies of deferred prescribing, for both upper respiratory tract infections and ENT infections, show 55% of patients given a deferred script did not use it (9).

Which Antibiotic?

BTS guidelines: amoxicillin as a first line choice, or a macrolide if allergic.

References

1. Symptoms, signs, and prescribing for acute lower respiratory tract illness. *British Journal of General Practice* 2001; 51: 177–181
2. Aetiology of respiratory tract infections: clinical assessment versus serological tests. *British Journal of General Practice* 2001; 51: 998–1000
3. Influence of patients' expectations on antibiotic management of acute lower respiratory tract illness in general practice: questionnaire study. *British Medical Journal* 1997; 315: 1211–1214
4. Quantitative systematic review of randomised controlled trials comparing antibiotic with placebo for acute cough in adults. *British Medical Journal* 1998; 316(7135): 906–910
5. Antibiotic prescribing and admissions with major suppurative

complications of respiratory tract infections: a data linkage study. *British Journal of General Practice* 2002; 52 (476): 187–193

6. Diagnosis and prognosis of lower respiratory tract infections: a cough is not enough. *British Journal of General Practice* 2001; 51: 174–177
7. Reducing reconsultations for acute lower respiratory tract illness with an information leaflet: a randomised controlled study of patients in primary care. *British Journal of General Practice* 1997;47: 719–722
8. Systematic review of randomised controlled trials of over the counter cough medicines for acute cough in adults. *British Medical Journal* 2002; 324: 329.
9. A randomised controlled trial of delayed antibiotic prescribing as a strategy for managing uncomplicated respiratory tract infection in primary care. *British Journal of General Practice* 2001: 51; 200–205

Answer 7 **As a result of an audit it has become clear that an excessive number of your patients fail to attend outpatient appointments after being referred by their GP. In a drive to improve access times you set up a working party to explore the causes of this. You wish the process to be evidence based.**

Outline how you would gather your evidence

- Define a question e.g. 'Why do patients fail to attend their appointments?'
- Identify and search resource areas:
  - Medline for world-wide literature search. Needs precise searching methodology. Local medical librarian may be of help.
  - Internet search of *British Medical Journal* archive, again with a clearly defined search terms and knowledge of system. May also try Royal College of General Practitioners website for references to back issues of *British Journal of General Practice*.
  - Textbooks. Local medical library may have access to useful textbooks, e.g. *Notes for the MRCGP*, which summarise research findings in some areas.
  - Word of mouth. Talking over with colleagues may open lines of inquiry. Potentially rewarding, but also potentially misleading.
- Agree screening process, e.g. priority for recent publications in respected peer reviewed journals (e.g. *British Medical Journal, British Journal of General Practice*) that are directly relevant. Consider hierarchy of evidence, with randomised controlled trials at top and case reports at bottom.
- Need to distinguish between qualitative and quantitative evidence. An area like this is likely to have a lot of qualitative evidence regarding causes and possibly quantitative evidence regarding possible solutions. For qualitative data randomised controlled trial is the gold standard, for qualitative data this is seldom practical.
- Screen results, selecting the most relevant that satisfy the above criteria.
- Summarise relevant data.

Comment on the strengths and weaknesses of the methodology of the study as presented in reference material 5.1a

Strengths

• Journal: Peer reviewed journal, relevant to UK general practice.
• Study design: Systematic approach studying all GP referrals avoids inclusion bias.
• Study population: Jarman score calculated from postcode, giving a quantifiable estimate of deprivation.
• Statistical analysis: Validated method of comparing populations. Clearly defined variables.
• All patients accounted for in data.

Weaknesses

• Study design: Prospective cohort study, potential for bias as GPs may be aware they are being studied and stress importance of attendance or alter referring habits. Running in parallel with a RCT will limit study design; unclear if this was on same patients, in which case potential bias from intervention.
• Studied all referrals from 26 GPs in 13 practices. Why so few GPs? Did some of the GPs in these practices object (source of possible inclusion bias)? How were they selected?
• Study population: Patients in Exeter may not be representative of patients in the rest of the UK, e.g. socio-economic and ethnic differences. This may limit applicability of study. Need baseline data on these variables. Referral rates calculated from referrals during study, may not be representative either because of GPs knowing they are being observed or seasonal variation, particularly as the study only looked at data from January to May.

Answer 8   Extracts from the results section of the paper referred to in the preceding question are given in reference material 5.2a.

What do you conclude from the results presented?

Characteristics of Non-Attenders Compared With Attenders and Cancellations

• The mean age, sex and interval between referral and appointment are all statistically significant as analysed in these results, with p values <0.05.
• The confidence interval for the sex distribution in the non-attenders is wide. A larger cohort may reduce the percentage of males closer to that of the attender group, which has narrower confidence intervals owing to its large size.
• The mean ages are markedly different with relatively narrow confidence intervals, suggesting this is a real difference, combined with a p value

<0.0001.
- The multivariable analysis of characteristics of non attendance suggest that male sex, age, Jarman score and interval to appointment are all statistically significant, with p values <0.05.

Characteristics of GPs

- The median interval between referral and appointment similarly has a statistically significant p value of <0.0001 but the confidence intervals are wide. A larger cohort would probably reduce this.
- The percentages for GPs by fundholding and MRCGP status are not significant, both with p values >0.05.
- The referral rate is borderline, with a p value of 0.05.

What other factors may explain the results seen?

There are several possible areas of confounding:
- The non-attendee cohort is relatively small, increasing the chance of misleading results.
- The conditions for which the non-attenders were referred with may have been self-limiting, e.g. rashes.
- Some of the non-attenders may have been treated with an acute presentation of their problem while waiting. Similarly they may have moved away from the area, died or had the operation carried out privately.
- Knowing the breakdown by speciality might provide more useful data, as all of the non-attenders may be clustered in one speciality with a particularly long waiting list skewing the average results.
- Geographical distance from hospital and transport options may also provide bias. Patients with their own transport are more likely to attend.
- Did the patients who failed to attend receive their appointment letters? Is there a problem with up-to-date records of addresses? Areas with high Jarman scores often have a high proportion of rented accommodation and itinerant populations.
- Another possibility is that the specialists or GPs may be giving preferential treatment to certain groups of patients with earlier appointments.

Answer 9   With reference to current evidence, discuss the effectiveness of the following interventions in management of stroke:

Stroke units

- Clinical Evidence: Stroke rehabilitation units reduce death and severe disability and increase independence at 1 year compared with general medical care.
- NSF for Elderly People and Stroke: Patients should have prompt access to integrated stroke care services. By 2004 PCTs will have to use protocols to identify, treat and refer stroke patients.

- Royal College of Physicians National Clinical Guidelines for Stroke suggest that everyone should be under the care of services specialising in stroke and rehabilitation. Should have a geographically defined unit, a co-ordinated multidisciplinary team with specialist expertise, provide education for staff, patients and carers, and have protocols for common problems. Do not need to be hospital-based.

Surgery

- Carotid endarterectomy for symptomatic carotid stenosis of greater than 70% shown to be beneficial (1).
- In the NASCET trial, the absolute risk reduction for ipsilateral ischaemic stroke after carotid endarterectomy was 28.9% (2).

Radiology

National Clinical Guidelines suggest diagnosis primarily clinical but urgent imaging should be considered if bleeding is suspected, if patients are deteriorating or trauma is suspected. All other patients should have brain imaging within 48 h.

Drug treatment

- Aspirin: The National Clinical Guidelines for Stroke suggest 300 mg aspirin should be given as soon as possible if haemorrhagic stroke unlikely on clinical grounds. This has been confirmed by meta-analysis (3).
- The HOPE study has shown that ramipril may reduce stoke in high risk patients, although the absolute risk reduction was small, approximately 1.5% (4).
- The Heart Protection Study showed that statins could reduce risk of stroke in both primary and secondary prevention (5).
- Warfarin may be effective particularly in patients with AF (Stroke prevention in AF trial) but is underused in practice. Trial efficacy has been shown to translate to effectiveness in the community (6).
- A Cochrane meta-analysis showed that patients receiving thrombolysis within 6 h of the onset of symptoms were less likely to die or become dependent than were controls, despite an increase in complications. Treatment within 3 h of onset of symptoms produced even better results (7).
- The LIFE (Losartan Intervention For Endpoint Reduction in Hypertension study) demonstrated a 25% reduction in risk of stroke compared to atenolol in high risk patients (8).

References

1. Benefit of carotid endarterectomy in patients with symptomatic moderate or severe stenosis. *New England Journal of Medicine* 1998; 339: 1415–1425
2. Risk, causes, and prevention of ischaemic stroke in elderly patients with

symptomatic internal-carotid-artery stenosis. *Lancet* 2001; 357(9263): 1154–1160

3. Collaborative meta-analysis of randomised trials of antiplatelet therapy for prevention of death, myocardial infarction, and stroke in high risk patients. *British Medical Journal* 2002; 324: 71–86

4. Use of ramipril in preventing stroke: double blind randomised trial. *British Medical Journal* 2002; 324: 699

5. Statins are the new aspirin, Oxford researchers say (News) *British Medical Journal* 2001; 323: 1145

6. Prospective cohort study to determine if trial efficacy of anticoagulation for stroke prevention in atrial fibrillation translates into clinical effectiveness. *British Medical Journal* 2000; 320: 1236–1239

7. Thrombolysis for acute ischaemic stroke. *Cochrane Database Systematic Review* 2000; (2): CD000213

8. Losartan Intervention for Endpoint Reduction in Hypertension study. *Lancet* 2000; 359: 1004–10

Answer 10   While looking at ways to improve the care of patients with epilepsy in your practice, you come across the paper 'A pragmatic randomized controlled trial of a prompt and reminder card in the care of people with epilepsy' (with permisison from *British Journal of General Practice* 2002; 52: 93–98; reference material 5.3a).

Comment on the strengths and weaknesses of the method described

Strengths

- The study is general practice-based, making it relevant to primary care management.
- The search criteria for identifying patients through a summary and medication search is appropriate to identify suitable patients.
- Practice selection was at random in the four areas, reducing the likelihood of inclusion bias.
- The intervention was a simple, standardised evidence-based prompt. This was designed to be easy to use in conjunction with medical records.
- Outcome measures were objective, allowing direct comparison, e.g. of seizure frequency.

Weaknesses

- Randomisation was done with a random number table. It is not clear how this was done and whether the stratification of practices before randomisation gave truly equivalent groups. Comparison data was not given between the three groups.
- Excluding those with learning disabilities makes the results less applicable to these patients, which is unfortunate since they may be the patients whose care is least satisfactory.
- The doctor-held paper prompt might be less useful in paperless practices

where the GPs do not routinely use paper notes.
- The length of the paper prompt might act as a disincentive during consultations when time is limited.
- The secondary outcomes of retrieval and completion rate of the card are not directly linked to improved quality of care, which was the aim of the trial.

Comment on the results of the trial (shown in Tables 1, 2 and 3 of reference material 5.3b)

- The data in Table 1 demonstrate that recording of seizure frequency in the notes is poor prior to the intervention, with only 37% of records including this data.
- After the intervention year the recording in the doctor-held record group had improved significantly (odds ratio 1.82, p = 0.003), but not the patient-held group.
- The self-reported seizure frequency data showed an increase in the numbers of patients in all three groups who were seizure free at the end of the intervention, but the increases were not statistically significant.
- The only statistically significant changes in Table 3 are that significantly more patients reported side effects in the intervention groups and that fewer patients reported satisfaction with GP information provision in the intervention groups.
- There were no differences in pharmacological management.

Comment on possible reasons for these results

- The increased recording by doctors may be explained by the Hawthorne effect, i.e. GPs who know they are being watched may concentrate more on data recording.
- These data suggest that the intervention increased recording at the expense of patient satisfaction, i.e. GPs may have been spending more time filling in record cards rather than listening to their patients. The aim of the intervention should be to improve care, not just improve record keeping.

Answer 11   Discuss the impact of deprivation on general practice.

Since Tudor Hart described the inverse care law many people have attempted to quantify the effect of deprivation on general practice. The most widely used tools are the Jarman and Townsend indices which use factors such as unemployment, single parent families and overcrowding.

Social Factors

- Higher unemployment, and if employed more likely to work shifts, with longer hours and less holiday and sick pay. May have less disposable income for prescriptions, heating, etc.
- Housing: Less likely to have central heating and inside toilets. More likely to be rented accommodation. More likely to be in industrial areas with

more pollution. Many rural areas may also be deprived. May be in areas of high crime.

- Access: More reliance on public transport or lifts from friends/family may result in more requests for home visits.
- Social stressors may result in more mental health problems, and certain underprivileged groups more likely in deprived areas, e.g. asylum seekers, ethnic minorities.
- Drug abuse more common.

Doctor Factors

- Demand is higher. More single mothers and people on low incomes.
- More 'difficult' problems, e.g. drugs, alcohol, psychological problems.
- Communication may be a problem where ethnic minorities may not speak English.
- Security may be an issue, e.g. an escort may be needed when doing home visits in areas of high crime.
- Burnout may be a problem in the face of seemingly insurmountable social problems, with high demand and low resources.

Patient Factors

- Higher morbidity and mortality at all ages. Accidents, especially in children, more common. Smoking more common, leading to lower life expectancy due to smoking-related disease, cancers, COPD, cardiovascular disease.
- Less access to preventive services.
- Lifestyle: Diet may be poor. Less access to sports facilities, and healthy lifestyle often a low priority.
- Education and literacy: Patient leaflets may not be understood, especially in ethnic minorities. Psychiatric morbidity is higher and may be unrecognised.
- Domestic violence and abuse more common.
- In areas of ethnic minorities, uncommon diseases may be seen, e.g. vitamin D deficient rickets, TB.
- Households less likely to have telephones, so there may be problems phoning for appointments.

Practice Factors

- May have lower income due to poor uptake of immunisations, smears, etc.
- Mobile population, require regularly updated records.
- Need good co-ordination with social services and health visitors.
- Recruitment and retention: Vacant posts impact on existing staff. Locums may be hard to find. PMS may help to address this with salaried posts and moving away from traditional incentive payments (e.g. smears) into more appropriate areas of need (e.g. drugs, asylum seekers).
- Practice leaflet need to be appropriate for patient language and literacy levels.

- Appointments: Approximately 50% higher consultation rate and chronic sickness rate is 40% higher in deprived areas. Walk-in surgeries or telephone triage may be more appropriate than traditional systems.
- Vandalism of premises may affect services. Crime including theft of prescription pads and burglary common. Will need good security systems in place and policies for dangerous or difficult patients.
- Health promotion clinics may require novel approaches to increase attendance.
- Interpreters may be required, or staff with language skills employed.
- Take educational abilities e.g. literacy into account when sending letters.

Wider Issues

- Holidays/study leave: May be hard to get locums to cover leave, affecting postgraduate education.
- PCT may need to employ locums to fill vacancies or cover holiday or leave.
- PCT may need novel approaches to managing demand, e.g. PMS contracts, health promotion clinics, walk-in centres etc.
- Some studies suggest bias in waiting times for secondary care services against deprived patients.

Answer 12   A 21-year-old girl and her boyfriend come for the morning-after pill. They both have Down's syndrome and attend a local daycare centre. What issues does this raise, and how would you proceed?

This situation poses a number of potential problems. The following should be borne in mind.

Consultation Issues

- Use appropriate language. Assume they are mentally competent unless there is evidence otherwise.
- Beware of conscious or subconscious prejudice.
- Do not assume she waives her confidentiality by bringing boyfriend in.

Ethical Issues

- Is she competent?
- Is she at risk?
- Has she fully consented to sex?

Doctor/Practice Issues

- Does this reflect failure of contraceptive advice?
- Are other areas of sexual health being neglected e.g. cervical smears, STD counselling?
- Has she not consulted before because she is always escorted by her parents?
- Has she been put off by previous experience of doctor's attitudes, e.g. patronism?

- Is there a problem with access to healthcare for patients with learning difficulties?

Medical Issues

- Is there any medical condition that makes pregnancy dangerous (e.g. congenital heart disease), or puts her at risk of venous thromboembolism?
- Could she be pregnant from earlier incidents?

Legal Issues

- Meticulous note keeping.
- If not competent, consider contacting defence organisation for advice trying to delay in providing emergency contraception.
- Be prepared for possible problems with parents.

Genetic Issues

High risk of Down's child. Can they understand genetic risk? Respect their opinions.

Management of the Problem

- Take a full sexual history: LMP (last menstrual period), dates of unprotected sexual intercourse, usual cycle. Using any contraception?
- Review previous medical history.
- Conduct a brief examination, e.g. CVS and BP.
- Consider need for pregnancy test if earlier exposures.

Immediate Treatment

- If no contraindications and treatment indicated, prescribe emergency contraception or consider emergency coil fitting.
- If not suitable for emergency contraception, seek advice of family planning clinic.
- Check her understanding throughout.
- Ensure she understands possible treatment failure.
- Plan follow-up, in particular future contraception, consider review for pregnancy test.

Future Treatment

- Need for effective contraception.
- Consider addressing other sexual health needs. e.g. smears?

Other Issues

- Assess provision of healthcare for patients with learning difficulties.
- If possibility of non-consensual sex, is there a lack of supervision at day care or at home?
- Are practice staff aware of confidentiality/consent issues?

Paper 6

Answer 1   Hannah, a normally fit and active 3-year-old, is brought to you by her parents. She is lethargic, dehydrated and smells ketotic. A fingerprick BM shows a blood glucose of 22. What are your aims, now and in the future?

You need to be sympathetic to parents, address their concerns and possible feelings of guilt. Try not to alarm or scare Hannah; talk to and examine her sensitively to put her at ease.

Immediate Management

Hannah almost certainly has diabetes. Immediate priorities are:
- Review history: Urinary frequency, appetite, weight loss, recent illness.
- Examination: Assess respiratory rate, signs of acidosis, dehydration.
- Management: Refer immediately to on-call paediatrician for rehydration, confirmation of diagnosis and insulin treatment.
- Explain likely diagnosis and need for investigation and initial treatment in hospital. Offer to telephone later to clarify any queries.

Short-term Management

Hannah and her family will need help and support, physically, financially and emotionally.
- Offer advice about support services, e.g. British Diabetic Association.
- Look out for guilt in parents, fear of diabetes in siblings and grief reactions as they realise Hannah has lost her excellent health. Look for denial and depression.
- Be aware of possible honeymoon period of low insulin requirements; family may challenge diagnosis.
- Initially most of care from paediatricians, but be prepared to share care later.
- Practice staff, e.g. health visitor and nurses, may need input to support family.

Long-term Management

- Aim for normal quality of life with minimal side effects and complications.
- Explain that good control may be at the expense of hypos. Prepare them for this if not done so in hospital (DCCT trial).
- Be aware of difficult times, e.g. exercise, illness, alcohol, school trips, adolescence, etc.
- Ensure nursery/school are happy and confident with care, possibly health

visitor to visit.
- Ensure she is on practice register. Importance of regular follow-up, e.g. retinal screening, kidney function.
- When she considers planning a family, ensure preconception counselling and consultant-led care.
- Advise on career implications, e.g. she cannot be an HGV driver.

Answer 2   'Growing old gracefully' – how can general practice meet the needs of elderly people?

- The percentage of people aged over 60 years in the UK is predicted to rise from 20 to 30% by 2031.
- The NSF for the Elderly aims to improve health and social care for these individuals with varied physical, practical and emotional needs.

Provision of Medical Care

- Age should not prejudice provision of treatment. Elderly people often have most to gain from preventive measures, e.g. anticoagulation in AF to reduce stroke.
- Healthcare advice, e.g. on weight, smoking, exercise, is never too late and often well received.
- Addressing mental health problems is important. Elderly people have a high incidence of depression, and suicide risk is underestimated. Bereavement may increase depression and social isolation. Need to actively seek mood disturbance and instigate appropriate treatment with minimum side effects (e.g. SSRIs), and have access to CPNs to support.
- Elder abuse is not uncommon, and the possibility must be considered.
- Ensure regular review – new targets to achieve over-75 checks.
- May need to actively call patients for review, e.g. by letter. If unable to attend, consider home visit by doctor, district nurse or health visitor.
- Appropriate use of medication: Physiological changes with ageing may affect side effects or doses.
- Avoid polypharmacy where possible. Regularly review need for medication, compliance and side effects. Drugs (e.g. benzodiazepines) may cause falls or accidents. Ensure practice has mechanisms to review repeat prescriptions.
- Ensure relationships with residential/nursing homes with access to help when needed. Potential benefits of educating staff, e.g. skin care, prevention of pressure sores, diabetic management.

Accessibility of Health Care

- Consider transport or disabilities affecting ability to attend surgeries. Consider provision of transport, e.g. for diabetic reviews, etc.
- Involve primary healthcare team, e.g. health visitor, for home and local day care visits.
- Provide information on services: Surgery contact numbers, NHS Direct, social services, elderly organisations, e.g. Help the Aged.

- Communication difficulties: Facilities for visually impaired (e.g. large print practice leaflet, etc.) and for hard of hearing (e.g. induction loops).
- Provision for physical disability, e.g. hand rails/ramps/lift at entrance. Comfortable spacious waiting area with minimum hazards and possibly raised chairs. Staff should be sensitive to patients who may need assistance.

Addressing Non-medical Issues

- Aim to reduce social isolation in those living alone with distant relatives unable to provide support. Practice staff need to provide information on resources, e.g. community buses for shopping, social/luncheon groups, daycare centres.
- Safety at home: Ensure provision of aids, e.g. walking frames, hand rails, home helps for cleaning/bathing assistance. Aim to maintain independent living in own home.
- Financial issues: Health visitors can help to complete benefit claims, etc.
- Respect autonomy: The competent have right to refuse help, others may need help (e.g. in dementia).
- Support for carers is often neglected. Their role can be very stressful and isolating. Ensure practice has record of carers. Consider carer support groups, be alert for signs of psychological distress.
- Ensure up-to-date records for elderly patients include next of kin, power of attorney and advance directives.

Implications of Improved Care

- Workload: Good care of elderly with long complicated consultations, regular reviews and home visits time consuming for whole of PHCT.
- Financial impact: Costs of adaptations to surgery premises, providing transport, and staff time. Ultimately these may be offset by more cost-effective and appropriate prescribing and reduced morbidity from falls, etc.
- Improved patient satisfaction: Should feel needs addressed, their health taken seriously and independence maintained.
- Will need regular audit to ensure achieving aims.
- Government requirements to implement the NSF have raised concerns that this represents more work for GPs to reduce hospital admissions. GPs may be required to provide 'intermediate/home care' which increases workload and may not be effective, or evidence-based. GPs may not have necessary skills.
- Needs considerable extra resources as demand will continue to increase as population grows.

Answer 3   The NSF for Elderly People and Stroke places new emphasis on the prevention and treatment of stroke. See reference material 6.1a, an extract from the paper 'Use of ramipril in preventing stroke: double blind randomized trial' (with permission from *British Medical Journal* 2002; 324; 699).

Comment on the methodology of the trial

- The study was a randomised double blind controlled trial. This is the gold standard study design.
- The study addressed a well formulated question: does ramipril prevent stroke in high risk patients? The study design was appropriate to answer this.
- The population was selected to be high risk for stroke. The exclusion criteria were reasonable and did not exclude too many patient groups.
- The intervention was similar to the standard use of ramipril in everyday practice, with monitoring of renal function, and the patients received no other intervention.
- All patients were put on to maximal ramipril dose. In practice this may not be tolerated by many patients. Data on the effectiveness of lower doses are not available, so the results may not be representative for patients on lower doses.
- Baseline characteristics are given but not split into intervention and control. Method of recruitment and randomization are not given, although a reference is made to earlier publications.
- Follow up was excellent with 99.9% follow up achieved.
- The outcomes were clinically appropriate endpoints of myocardial infarction, stroke or cardiovascular death. Stroke was diagnosed by CT where possible and an adjudication committee decided on diagnoses using records. Recovery was judged according to a standardised six point scale, reducing recall and observer bias.

Comment on the results in Table1 of reference material 6.1b

- The results show a reduction in total strokes from 4.9% to 3.4%, a relative risk reduction of 32%.
- The reductions here are 1.0 % to 0.4% (RR reduction 61%) for fatal strokes and 3.9% to 3.0% (RR reduction 24%) for non-fatal strokes.
- The reductions are seen in both ischaemic and non-ischaemic strokes.
- The table does not give p values, but the confidence intervals for all of these are consistent with a positive effect except for non-ischaemic stroke where the confidence intervals cross 1.
- These results appear to support the hypothesis that ramipril reduces the incidence of stroke.

Comment on the statement from the conclusion 'Widespread use of an angiotensin converting enzyme inhibitor such as ramipril in patients at high risk of stroke is likely to have a major impact on public health'

- The results of this study, while showing impressive relative risk reductions are less impressive when absolute risk reductions are considered.
  - For total strokes the ARR is 1.5 %, i.e. a number needed to treat of 67 to prevent 1 stroke.
  - For non-fatal strokes the ARR is 0.9%, i.e. a NNT of 111 to prevent 1 non-fatal stroke.

– For fatal strokes the ARR is 0.6%, i.e. a NNT of 166 to prevent 1 fatal stroke.
- The side effects of ramipril are not insignificant, with a small number developing worsening renal impairment as a result.
- The funds necessary to implement the prescribing of ramipril in all patients at high risk might be better spent in funding rehabilitation services.

Answer 4   **The practice receptionist points out that there seem to be a large number of patients not attending appointments. What do you need to consider when looking at this problem?**

- Patients missing appointments waste a considerable amount of resources and contributes to long access times.
- The first step is to assess the scale of the problem by auditing non-attenders. Involve receptionists, e.g. record over a 1-month period. Determine acceptable levels given the practice demographics (e.g. level of deprivation).
- What groups of patients appear to miss appointments?
- Do the numbers vary between different partners or with locums?

What Factors Need to be Considered with Regard to DNA Rates?

Patient Issues

- May be legitimate reasons for not attending – family/work crisis, car breakdown, no access to telephone.
- Misinterpretation of time when booking – e.g. not written down, or forgotten.
- Limited access early in illness may lead to recovery or seeking help elsewhere, e.g. A & E or walk-in centre.
- With sensitive or embarrassing problems a patient may lose courage to attend or be put off by questioning from receptionists.
- Fail to realise importance of cancelling to free up spaces.
- Some patients are embarrassed to cancel – easier just not to turn up.
- Some patients are just unreliable.

Doctor Issues

- You may welcome a few non-attenders. The space provides an opportunity to catch up if running behind, make phone calls and have a coffee.
- You may feel angry about the waste of time and lack of courtesy to cancel.
- High non-attendance rates increase waiting times, affecting other patients.
- For important consultations, e.g. to discuss abnormal test results, chasing patients by phone or letter is more time-consuming and frustrating.
- Non-attendance may be related to your consulting style, unnecessary

follow-ups, or poor communication with patients.
* You may habitually run late, causing patient frustration.

Practice Nurse/Physiotherapist Issues

* Similar issues to doctors. Appointments often longer, even more time wasted.
* Patients may see nurse appointments as second best and fail to attend.

Reducing Numbers

* Patient questionnaires may explore cause and suggest strategies to reduce missed appointments.
* Posters highlighting importance of cancelling appointments if patient can't attend. Clearly state in practice leaflet.
* Particular groups or families who frequently fail to attend may be identified and reminded, but this is time consuming.
* Consider warning or removal from list for patients who frequently fail to attend.
* Issue written confirmation of appointment time when booking
* Improve access – aim for 24/48 h, look at Advanced Access strategies.
* Review follow-up appointments. Are they all necessary? Pass responsibility to patient to re-attend if not improving.
* Increase appointment time to e.g. 15 minutes – may improve patient satisfaction and reduce re-attendance.
* Re-audit after changes implemented.

Local Issues

* Do local practices have similar problems? Are more GPs needed?
* Is access in tune to local needs? Offer variety of sources to access medical help at convenient times, e.g. walk-in centre, more nurse-led minor illness clinics. May need targeted funding.
* Danger that easier access may increase demand.
* Non-attendance in primary care may be mirrored in secondary care, affecting access here.
* Consider community media campaign highlighting impact of non-attendance on resources for NHS and waiting lists.

Answer 5   A 30-year-old woman with a BMI of 32 comes to see you requesting a prescription for slimming drugs which she read about in a magazine. What issues does this consultation raise?

Obesity is a major health problem in developed countries, increasing the risk of conditions such as diabetes mellitus, ischaemic heart disease and joint disease. These patients are a significant drain on health service resources.

Issues raised by this Consultation

Patient Issues

- Why has she presented now? Does she or a family member have an obesity-related illness? Is she experiencing relationship or work problems? Is she happy with weight but has been encouraged to attend by a partner, relative or boss?
- Does she have poor self-esteem or psychological illness, e.g. depression? Is she being victimised about her weight?
- Any hidden agendas, e.g. concern about polycystic ovaries or infertility?
- What are her ideas about weight loss and diet? Has she tried other diets or slimming clubs?
- Does she have friends who have tried medications? Are her expectations realistic?

Doctor Issues

- Sensitive issue. Importance of rapport. Be non-judgemental with regular follow-up.
- Exclude secondary causes (e.g. hypothyroidism, Cushing's) and co-morbidity (e.g. BP, diabetes).
- Question about other risk factors, e.g. smoking, alcohol. Is she on the pill? Obesity is a relative contraindication.
- Aim to explore her understanding of obesity and its risks. What interventions has she tried before? May benefit from referral to dietician.
- If considering medication explain that she needs to achieve initial weight loss with diet alone, exclude contraindications, counsel about side effects, monitoring and length of treatment.
- Potentially a long and stressful consultation with implications for time management.
- Any learning needs regarding obesity management and drug treatments?
- Need to be aware of NICE guidance on prescribing criteria for orlistat and sibutramine.
- Doctor prejudices may affect consultation, e.g. see obesity as lack of self-control and the patient's own responsibility rather than a medical issue.

Practice Issues

- Increasingly common reason for consultation – often long, frequent appointments which use a lot of GP time.
- Often involve practice nurses for weight monitoring and dietary advice. Nurses need education on obesity management.
- Resources should be available in the practice for patients, e.g. leaflets, diet sheets and videos.
- Consider setting up a patient support group, but may have time and resource implications.

- If this is an area of interest for partner or nurse consider establishing dedicated obesity clinic.

Wider Issues

- Are anti-obesity drugs expensive 'lifestyle drugs' which burden the cash limited NHS?
- Obesity is a major health problem, using valuable NHS resources.
- Should PCTs fund community dieticians, community-led support groups, subsidy for membership of gyms, etc.?
- Controversies over efficacy and safety, e.g. concerns about NICE guidance.
- Issues regarding society's attitude to weight in general, the media portrayal of thinness as ideal.
- Should we lobby government and the food industry to improve quality and pricing of foods?
- Aim to educate children and improve quality of school meals, and make exercise attractive, accessible and affordable.

Answer 6 With reference to recent literature, discuss the use of the following in primary care:

Nurse practitioners

The NHS plan aims to extend the role of nurses and to encourage all professionals to work together. Nurses have been seen as an ideal solution to staff shortages in general practice.

Are Nurse Practitioners Effective?

A systematic review (1) suggests patients are more satisfied with care from nurse practitioners than doctors, with no difference in health outcomes. Nurse practitioners provide longer consultations and carry out more investigations than doctors. Most research has looked at same day appointments for minor illness, which is only a limited part of a doctor's role. Some of the trials are of questionable relevance to the NHS since qualifications and roles vary considerably throughout the world, as does the use of the term nurse practitioner.

Are they Useful for Emergency Appointments?

For same day appointments Venning found clinical care and health service costs were similar, and concluded that if nurse practitioners were able to maintain the benefits while reducing their return consultation rate or shortening consultation times, they could be more cost effective than GPs (2).

Are they Useful for Telephone Triage?

Lattimer et al. (3) found nurse triage in out-of-hours care halved the number of cases dealt with by GPs and was at least as safe as existing services. Nurse telephone consultation replaced telephone advice given by a doctor and led to reductions in both home visits and surgery attendances out of hours.

Are Nurse Minor Illness Clinics Effective?

- In a randomised controlled trial Shum (4) found that in 73% of consultations no doctor input was needed. Again, patients were more satisfied with their consultations with nurses than their consultations with doctors
- Clinical outcomes were similar, while nurses took an average of 8 minutes per patient compared to 10 minutes for GPs.
- A *British Medical Journal* editorial (5) concluded that on average, nurses have longer consultations, arrange more investigations and follow up, provide more information, and give more satisfaction than general practitioners. Primary care nurses are not cheaper than general practitioners, but they are as safe in managing self-limiting illnesses.

Community pharmacists

The burden of repeat prescribing is ever expanding, and it has been suggested that community pharmacists can manage this. The proposed benefits include safer prescribing, with reduction in side effects and drug interactions, cheaper prescribing bills and time savings for GPs.

Are Consultations with a Pharmacist to Review Repeat Medications Effective?

A randomised controlled trial found more drug changes and lower prescribing costs than normal care plus a much higher review rate. Use of healthcare services by patients was not increased (6).

Can Pharmacists Reduce Prescribing Costs?

- A paper comparing a community pharmacist managed repeat prescription system with usual care found that 66% of patients did not require their full quota of drugs, saving 18% of the drug budget. Significantly more compliance problems, side effects, adverse reactions and interactions were also identified (7).
- A trial of educational outreach from community pharmacists concluded this was only effective in small practices (8).

Do the Costs Outweigh The Savings?

- A trial showed that savings exceed costs (9).
- Trial data involving enthusiastic well-motivated pharmacists who are being observed as part of a trial may not transfer to the wider health service. Pilot schemes are under way in 40 PCTs to test this.

References

1. Systematic review of whether nurse practitioners working in primary care can provide equivalent care to doctors. *British Medical Journal* 2002; 324: 819–823
2. Randomised controlled trial comparing cost effectiveness of general practitioners and nurse practitioners in primary care. *British Medical Journal* 2000; 320: 1048–1053
3. Safety and effectiveness of nurse telephone consultation in out of hours primary care: randomised controlled trial. *British Medical Journal* 1998; 317: 1054–1059
4. Nurse management of patients with minor illnesses in general practice: multicentre, randomised controlled trial. *British Medical Journal* 2000; 320: 1038–1043
5. Nursing and the future of primary care. *British Medical Journal* 2000; 320: 1020–1021
6. Randomised controlled trial of clinical medication review by a pharmacist of elderly patients receiving repeat prescriptions in general practice. *British Medical Journal* 2001; 323: 1340
7. Repeat prescribing: a role for community pharmacists in controlling and monitoring repeat prescriptions. *British Journal of General Practice* 2000; 50: 271–275
8. Controlled trial of pharmacist intervention in general practice: the effect on prescribing costs. *British Journal of General Practice* 1999; 49: 717–720
9. Controlled trial of pharmacist intervention in general practice: the effect on prescribing costs. A randomised controlled trial of the effect of educational outreach by community pharmacists on prescribing in UK general practice. *British Journal of General Practice* 1999; 49: 717–720

Answer 7   Discuss the evidence relating to the following in the diagnosis and management of dementia:

Assessment

• The North of England Evidence Based Guidelines (1) suggest formal assessment using the MMTS, as subjective complaints of memory loss are not a good indicator.
• Routine blood and urine tests should be done and Lewy body dementia excluded, as neuroleptics are hazardous in this group.
• Depression may be both a cause and a consequence of symptoms and should be actively sought and treated.
• In cases of sudden behavioural change, causes (e.g. physical or social) should be sought. Falls are common.

Drug treatments

Gingko

A systematic review of double blind randomised controlled trials (reported in *Clinical Evidence* (2)) found gingko improved cognitive function and is well tolerated. *Bandolier* (3) looked at the evidence and concluded it was effective with a NNT of 7. It also has antiplatelet effects (4).

Cholinesterase Inhibitors

- Clinical evidence suggests donepezil is effective, and rivastigmine likely to be so.
- NICE guidance for these drugs and galantamine advises that they should be available on the NHS for mild to moderate Alzheimer's, for patients with a MMSE > 12/30, should only be initiated by a specialist and should only continue if MMSE > 12.
- *Cochrane Review* (5) 2000 suggested that they were effective in improving cognitive function and global clinical state, but not patient-rated quality of life.
- Rivastigmine has been shown to increase cognitive scores and carer-rated quality of life (6).
- A *British Medical Journal* editorial discussing the NICE guidance also points out that the development of effective treatments will lead to a paradigm shift towards treatment rather than palliation and acknowledges the NICE guidance suggestion that secondary care services such as memory clinics need to be improved (7).

Statins

Several studies show a protective effect from statins (8).

Selegiline

Clinical Evidence (9) states that there is some RCT evidence for selegiline for improving cognitive function.

Social care

A study compared care in the NHS and the private sector. Of 500 patients studied, none was receiving appropriate care and an average of 12 minutes a day was spent in constructive activities. Erroneous attitudes among staff were partly to blame (10).

References

1. North of England evidence based guidelines development project: guideline for the primary care management of dementia. *British Medical Journal* 1998; 317: 802–808
2. Effect of treatments on cognition *Clinical Evidence 7* (August 2002). Section: Mental health, Dementia
3. Dementia – diagnosis and treatment. *Bandolier* 1998: 48; 2–3
4. Gingko biloba for dementia. *Clinical Drug Investigation* 1999; 17: 301–308
5. Donepezil for mild and moderate Alzheimer's disease *The Cochrane*

Library, Issue 3, 2002

6. Efficacy and safety of rivastigmine in patients with Alzheimer's disease: international randomised controlled trial. *British Medical Journal* 1999; 318: 633–640
7. Drugs for Alzheimer's disease. *British Medical Journal* 2001; 323: 123–124
8. Study adds to evidence that statins reduce risk of Alzheimer's disease. *British Medical Journal* 2002; 324: 936
9. Effects of treatments on cognition *Clinical Evidence 7* (August 2002). Section: Mental health, Dementia
10. Quality of care in private sector and NHS facilities for people with dementia: cross sectional survey. *British Medical Journal* 2001; 323: 426–427

Answer 8   Discuss how doctors can identify their learning needs.

- Identification of learning needs forms the basis for personal learning plans, recommended both for personal learning and a requirement for reappraisal.
- PLPs are individual. Lecture-based teaching suits some, while others learn best in small groups or self-directed learning. PLPs allow the use of variety of learning styles to best suit personal style and needs.

Identification of Learning Needs

Consultation-based Methods

- Patients' unmet needs (PUNS) and doctor's educational needs (DENS).
- Clinical problems or queries prompt self-directed learning, e.g. looking up specific facts about a condition, its management, investigation and treatment.
- Patient follow-up may highlight failed treatment or poor understanding of disease process. Patient questions may expose weaknesses, which may be difficult for the doctor. Bluffing, holding or honesty are all techniques used to gain time for information gathering.
- These enquiries may be prompted by the internet or media. Some doctors may resent this, while others embrace it as part of modern medicine.
- Joint surgeries allow us to learn how our colleagues manage their patients and allow sharing of consultation styles.
- Video consultations may highlight consultation problems and allow third party opinion.
- Patient questionnaires may demonstrate clinical and consultation learning needs.

Practice-based Methods

- Conventional audit may show deficiencies in process of care and outcomes.
- Significant event audit may highlight deficiencies in systems and learning

needs, e.g. missed diagnosis. These may then stimulate conventional audit to prevent further similar events. Sharing of positive and negative experiences, and reflection in a safe environment, make this a valuable tool.
- Staff feedback and practice meetings may allow all staff to point out areas of weakness in the others knowledge base.
- Practice appraisals: Comparison with other practices may allow learning needs on a practice and personal level to be identified.

Learning Needs Identified by Patients

- Complaints may reveal learning needs, e.g. in delayed diagnosis as well as consultation needs and deficiencies in the process of care.
- Patient satisfaction surveys: Provide confidential feedback on doctor's communication skills, attitudes and time-keeping.

Other Sources

- Guidelines may differ from doctor's current management and stimulate research.
- Journals may highlight new ideas, which may stimulate learning. Some magazines e.g. *Pulse*, have update sections which refresh and appraise knowledge in certain areas.
- The internet may present new avenues of information for both doctors and patients, although these may need critical appraisal.
- The Prodigy system may highlight alternative management options in researching learning needs.
- Computer-based learning and assessment (e.g. the PEP CD) and internet distance learning appraisals (e.g. MCQs) may highlight areas for attention.
- Educational courses advertised in the medical press may be of relevance and assist learning.
- Visits to neighbouring or beacon practices may stimulate critical appraisal of our own work.

Ethical Issues

- We have an ethical obligation to keep up-to-date, although we have autonomy in how we learn.
- Confidentiality issues need to be clarified, e.g. with significant event audits.

Answer 9 One of your practice nurses wishes to go on a course on screening for prostate cancer. What issues does this raise and how would you address her request?

Prostate cancer is the second commonest cause of male cancer death, with significant effects on quality of life. 60% of cases are metastatic at diagnosis. There is no consensus on whether screening or early aggressive treatment reduces mortality or morbidity.

This request raises several important issues.

Why Now?

- Why has she made the request?
- Significant event involving a missed diagnosis?
- A personal learning need in male health, e.g. stimulated by family or friend affected?
- Course advertised locally or run by the local PCO?
- Burnout: Do courses allow a break from the practice?
- Are patients she sees in the practice asking her for screening?

Review Current Practice

- Counselling: who does this? Is it the doctors or the practice nurse team?
- How is screening currently done? Digital examination or PSA or both?
- Over-75 health checks: Is there a need to discuss screening at these reviews?
- Review current guidelines. NICE guidance on referral for prostatism suggests offering men a PSA test with adequate counselling, but there is no national screening programme. No agreement on the best test but recent evidence suggests PSA should be combined with digital rectal examination.

Course Issues

- Who is running it? Drug-sponsored or run by a local postgraduate centre?
- Any likely bias?

Financial Issues

- Cost of the course
- Costs of covering study leave or locum nurse
- Increased investigations and referrals may result from positive screening results.

Practice Issues

Employment Issues

- Study leave: Should be included in nurse contracts.
- Need budget for study leave, either allocated to individuals or shared with other staff.
- Equity issues: Is study leave shared equally? Colleagues will have to cover for absence and may compete for leave, e.g. for holidays. Is there a need for prioritising study leave based on the benefit to the practice?

Training Issues

- Do the partners feel the course is necessary? Consider inviting a local urologist to discuss the issues with the practice staff as a whole.
- Digital rectal examination: Who will do it? Will course attendance by the nurse save GP appointments or create additional ones for rectals?

- Is there a well man clinic? Is this a good time to consider starting one if the nurse has identified a need? Does the practice have a high number of elderly patients? Consider offering screening at the over-75 health check.
- Any PCT interest? Screening may increase secondary care referrals. Will the PCT fund the course?

Ethical Issues

- Resources: Until screening is shown to be effective is it justified?
- Non-malificence/beneficence: Harm may be prevented if screening detects disease which can be treated, but increased anxiety and side effects from treatment and investigation in false positives may cause harm.
- Autonomy: Informed patients should be able to request or refuse screening.
- Consent: Informed consent, addressing the implications of a positive or negative result.
- Justice: Any screening programme should be offered to all the population to be targeted, not reserved for the worried, well-informed well.

Answer 10   With regard to child health in primary care, comment on the following areas of controversy, giving evidence to support your views:

Attention deficit hyperactivity disorder

Diagnosis

- Studies suggest 3–5% of school age children are affected (1).
- There is no validated diagnostic test. Core symptoms of inattention, hyperactivity, and impulsivity are also normal behavioural traits present in unaffected children. Need to be present in a variety of social situations.
- Diagnosis should be made by specialists.

Treatment

- 1.5 million prescriptions for stimulants in UK in 1995.
- RCT comparison of medication, intensive behavioural treatment, medication plus intensive behavioural treatment, and standard community care showed significantly greater improvement among groups that were given medication (2).
- Systematic review concludes stimulants are effective in the short term, are more effective than placebo, compare well with each other, and seem to be more effective than tricyclics and non-drug treatments (3).
- Treatment with methylphenidate may cause weight gain and hypertension. Full blood count needs checking regularly (BNF).

Neonatal screening

Deafness

- The Newborn Hearing Screening Programme to screen newborn babies

with otoacoustic emission (OAE) testing has recently been introduced. False positives occur due to transient middle ear obstruction. Auditory brainstem response testing is carried out on babies who fail OAE.
- A retrospective review suggests prevalence of deafness rises with age and that relying solely on neonatal screening will miss 50–90% of children who develop deafness by the age of 9 (4).
- Hence there is a need for surveillance of school age children in addition to neonatal screening.

Congenital Dislocation of the Hip

- A national orthopaedic surveillance scheme found that the incidence of a first operation for congenital dislocation of the hip (CDH) in the UK was 0.78 per 1,000 live births. CDH had not been detected by routine screening in 222 (70%) of 318 children reported to the scheme (5).
- Other strategies, e.g. ultrasound, may produce unacceptably high numbers of false positives with resultant side effects of unnecessary splinting.

Cataracts

A survey found only 47% of children diagnosed with congenital cataract had been diagnosed through standard childhood surveillance, with 33% not diagnosed until after their 1st birthday, increasing risk of permanent visual impairment (6).

References

1. Evidence and belief in ADHD. *British Medical Journal* 2000; 321: 975–976
2. A 14-month randomised clinical trial of treatment strategies for attention-deficit/hyperactivity disorder. The MTA Cooperative Group. Multimodal treatment study of children with ADHD. *Archives of General Psychiatry* 1999; 56: 1073–1086
3. *A review of therapies for attention-deficit/hyperactivity disorder.* Ottawa: Canadian Coordinating Office for Health Technology Assessment, 1998
4. Prevalence of permanent childhood hearing impairment in the United Kingdom and implications for universal neonatal hearing screening: questionnaire based ascertainment study. *British Medical Journal* 2001; 323: 536
5. Surgery for congenital dislocation of the hip in the UK as a measure of outcome of screening. *Lancet* 1998; 351: 1149–52
6. National cross sectional study of detection of congenital and infantile cataract in the United Kingdom: role of childhood screening and surveillance. *British Medical Journal* 1999; 318: 362–365

Answer 11   What are the problems encountered in studying therapies in arthritis?

- Problems may arise in identifying clinically relevant but objective outcome measures. Pain may be affected by many other variables as well as arthritis activity, such as depression, and this may act as a confounder.
- Symptoms often wax and wane, and apparent resolution may be coincidence or due to a therapy under investigation.
- Clinical outcomes such as joint replacement may be decided on subjectively and this decision may be dependent on local resources, e.g. where there are long waiting lists for surgery it is less likely to be offered to patients.

Comment on the methodology described in reference material 6.2a

- The trial was a randomised double blind placebo controlled trial, the gold standard clinical trial.
- Patients were included if they met formal diagnostic criteria for osteoarthritis (OA), reducing the risk of confounding by other conditions (e.g. rheumatoid arthritis).
- X-rays were assessed automatically by a computer, avoiding bias in assessing outcomes.
- The use of x-ray changes is a surrogate outcome and may not reflect symptom frequency, however this was combined with symptom assessment by a validated system, the WOMAC score.
- The study population size was calculated in advance to give sufficient power. The participants were selected from the outpatient clinic of a specialist centre, so they may not be representative of the general population e.g. they may have severe osteoarthritis unresponsive to normal treatments. It is unclear how they were recruited, raising the possibility of inclusion bias, e.g. only certain groups being invited to join the study.
- Exclusion criteria included BMI > 30. Many patients with OA will fall into this group and hence the results may not be applicable to the general practice population of patients.
- Randomisation was computerised, with sealed envelopes to blind the participants and examiners, avoiding inclusion/exclusion bias.
- The analysis was done on an intention-to-treat basis, making the results applicable to a clinical setting.
- The study was conducted over a 3-year period, sufficient to detect any effects.

Comment on the results in Tables 2 and 3 of reference material 6.2b

Table 2

When patients taking the treatment for three years are compared with those taking placebo, there was no significant reduction in mean joint space or minimum joint space in the glucosamine group, with confidence intervals crossing 0. The placebo group had a statistically significant decrease, and the difference of 0.38mm was significant with 95% confidence intervals of –0.17 to 0.32, p = 0.038. Similar results were obtained for minimum joint space narrowing.

These statistically significant results persisted when intention-to-treat analysis was carried out, with p values < 0.05 for both mean and minimum joint space.

Table 3

These results confirm a statistically significant difference of 34.1% (6.4 to 61.8) p = 0.016 for patients completing the trial and 21.6% (3.5 to 39.6) p = 0.020 for intention-to-treat. These confirm a benefit for Womac scores in patients taking glucosamine.

Answer 12   See reference material 6.3a, an extract from the paper 'The effect of GP telephone triage on numbers seeking same day appointments' (with permission from *British Journal of General Practice* 2002; 52: 390–392).

In terms of relevance to managing demand in UK general practice, discuss the methodology and results of this study

Population

• The study was carried out in a market town in a practice with a list size of 7,200. It is unclear whether it was the only practice in town or whether there was a minor illness unit in the town. Analysis of workload at these sites during the same period may show that patients offered telephone advice only simply went elsewhere for a face-to-face consultation.
• Jarman scores are given, but not ethnic mix. In areas with large ethnic communities who may not speak English as a first language, the policy may be less effective.
• There is no mention of the age distribution of the population. This may affect the acceptability of the intervention. Younger patients may prefer to have telephone advice, avoiding a consultation, whereas the elderly may be the opposite.

Doctors

• No attempt was made to assess the satisfaction of the doctors with this form of triage. Many doctors find telephone triage stressful and prefer face-to-face consultations, particularly with children and patients they do not know.
• Do the partners have personal lists? Anecdotal evidence suggests patients

are happier receiving, and doctors happier giving, telephone advice to
people that they know.
- Was all the triage done by the duty doctor or by each doctor triaging their
own patients?
- It is difficult to assess the impact of the drop in demand since only a
percentage reduction is given rather than an actual figure for reduction in
appointments or hours consulting saved. The time demands of telephone
triage are approximately one hour a day. Does this reduce appointments
by more than an hour a day? If not, the savings may be illusory.

Assessment

- Did the doctors know when they were going to have the patient
satisfaction survey done? This may have introduced bias by them
modifying their behaviour.
- The method states that a patient satisfaction survey was sent to all patients
who received a telephone call over a 1-month period. The results state
that a 74% response rate with 111 responses was achieved, i.e. 150
questionnaires were sent out. The results go on to state that during the
second half of the study, the average monthly call number was around
600. Did the workload increase fourfold between the two sampling
periods? If so, the GP activity log should have been conducted on the
same period as the satisfaction survey. Alternatively, did each person ring
for a same day appointment 4 times in the month, negating the benefits of
the intervention in reducing demand? A third explanation is that the
surveys were sent out to all callers over a 1-week period, not 1 month as
reported in the paper.
- What was the effect on demand for routine appointments? Patients may
have learnt that to be seen they need to ask for a routine rather than same
day appointment. Increased demand for routine appointments may
cancel out any savings made in emergency appointments.
- No attempt was made to compare doctor triage with nurse triage. GPs are
an expensive commodity to use for telephone triage. It may be that nurses
could provide a similar service at lower cost.

Financial costs

- Any other financial costs? Tying up an outside line for triage for 1 hour a
day may block incoming calls, requiring further investment in hardware.
- Did prescribing change before and after the intervention? Prescriptions
were offered in 22.4 % of consultations. A large proportion of these
presumably were for antibiotics, telephone prescribing of which is
frowned on by the Standing Advisory Committee. Increased prescribing
costs may remove any benefit in reduced appointments.

Abbreviations

ACE	acetylcholine esterase	INR	International Normalized Ratio
AF	atrial fibrillation	IOS	items of service
ARR	absolute risk reduction	LFT	liver function test
BMA	British Medical Association	LH	luteinising hormone
BMI	body mass index	LMC	local medical committee
BNF	British National Formulary	LMP	last menstrual period
BP	blood pressure	LV	left ventricle
CBT	cognitive behavioural therapy	MDU	Medical Defence Union
CDH	congenital dislocation of the hip	MI	myocardial infarction
CHImp	Commission for Health Improvement	MMR	measles, mumps and rubella vaccination
CNS	central nervous system		
COCP	combined oral contraceptive pill	MMTS	mini mental test score
COPD	chronic obstructive pulmonary disease	MS	multiple sclerosis
CPN	community psychiatric nurse	NICE	National Institute for Clinical Excellence
CVS	central venous system		
DENS	doctor's educational needs	NNT	number needed to treat
DEXA	dual energy x-ray absorptiometry	NSAID	non-steroidal anti-inflammatory drug
DM	diabetes mellitus	NSF	National Service Framework
DNA	deoxyribonucleic acid	OA	osteoarthritis
DOH	Department of Health	OAE	otoacoustic emission
DSM IV	APA *Diagnostic and Statistical Manual*, 4th edition	PACT	Prescribing Analysis and Cost
		PCG	primary care group
DVLA	Driver and Vehicle Licensing Authority	PCO	primary care organisation
DVT	deep venous thrombosis	PCT	primary care trust
ECG	electrocardiogram	PHCT	primary health care trust
ENT	ear, nose and throat	PLP	personal learning plan
ESR	erythrocyte sedimentation rate	PMS	Personal Medical Services
FBC	full blood count	PPI	proton pump inhibitor
FEV_1	forced expiratory volume in 1 second	PSA	prostate specific antigen
FSH	follicle stimulating hormone	PTSD	post-traumatic stress disorder
GI	gastrointestinal	PUNS	patients' unmet needs
GMC	General Medical Council	PVS	persistent vegetative state
GMS	General Medical Services	RCN	Royal College of Nurses
GORD	gastro-oesophageal reflux disease	SERM	selective oestrogen receptor modulator
GUM	genito-urinary medicine	SLE	systemic lupus erythematosis
HDL	high density lipoproteins	SSRI	selective serotonin re-uptake inhibitor
HIV	human immunodeficiency virus	STD	sexually transmitted disease
HRT	hormone replacement therapy	TFT	thyroid function test
IBS	irritable bowel syndrome	TIA	transient ischaemic attack
IHD	ischaemic heart disease	WHO	World Health Organization

Index